GOD'S CAREGIVERS

WHAT IS THE MESSAGE OF FAITH THAT "GOD'S CAREGIVERS" HAS TO OFFER?

"GOD'S CAREGIVERS—A Journey of Faith" is the story of a family that embarks upon a sacred journey. Their odyssey starts with the birth, in 1962, of identical male twins, seriously afflicted with spinal tumors, a result of severe cases of neuro-fibroma-tosis, a progressive disease that can disfigure, disable, and/or kill. As our then minister wrote, "You are my heroes, because you're doing God's work".

For over thirty-nine years, it has been, and is now, an ongoing case of abiding love and care, tendered by us as their parents and driven by a combination of love, obligation, necessity, and faith.

Along the way, those both in and out of churches that were not afraid to care helped ease the trauma of red tape and bureaucracies.

Our sons have made it clear that God's world is far from perfect, but their faith, limited though it may be and sorely tested, coupled with our tenacity, makes "GOD'S CAREGIVERS" a true "Journey of Faith".

Robert and Jane Weeber

God's Caregivers

A Journey of Faith

Robert V. Weeber

Writers Club Press
San Jose New York Lincoln Shanghai

God's Caregivers
A Journey of Faith

Writers Club Press
an imprint of iUniverse, Inc.

For information address:
iUniverse, Inc.
5220 S. 16th St., Suite 200
Lincoln, NE 68512
www.iuniverse.com

Any mention of an individual by name is intended to be informational only and in no way intended to reflect critically on that person's character or job performance.

ISBN: 0-595-21698-6

Printed in the United States of America

In Memoriam

Robert Vincent (Bobby, as he liked to be called) Weeber was born July 12, 1962, in Jacksonville, Florida, along with his identical brother, Nicky. Both were born with a condition later diagnosed as neuro-fibromatosis, originally known as Von Recklinghausen's Disease, after a German doctor who first identified it. It is a progressive ailment, characterized by tumors (usually, but not always, benign) that can disfigure, disable and kill.

In his early teens, Bobby underwent a spinal fusion operation to correct a scoliosis condition. Also, multiple operations by some of the finest neurosurgeons in the world, to decompress the spinal cord and remove tumors that had shut down his nervous system. The last operation, at Duke University Medical Center in 1990, left him permanently paralyzed from his hips down. After a brief spell at MUSC Rehab Center in Charleston and at a local nursing home, Bobby had been at home ever since.

His special interest was in corresponding with the New York and Hollywood TV stars, typing letters and fantasy biographical episodes about his ministers, his barber, and favorite home-health aide, in collaboration with his brother. Although he missed out on much that life offered most of his peers, he lived with courage and dignity and in so doing, touched more lives positively than most of us will do in lifetimes that run three times as long.

A succession of cats was an outlet for his concern for pets. His love of TV and a collection of videocassettes, plus typing, were his links to the "outside" world.

He kept informed with tabloids and daily newspapers and was articulate, intelligent, and a knowledgeable conversationalist. A pleasure for those who took the time to know, to understand, and to appreciate.

Bobby graduated from York Suburban High School, in York, Penn. in 1982. He did volunteer service at York Hospital, York, Penn., during his high school years and afterwards. Confirmed as a member of Eastminster Presbyterian Church, York, Penn., he transferred his letter upon arriving in Summerville and was a member of the Summerville Presbyterian Church.

Bobby passed away April 3, 1993, with the same dignity and grace that he exhibited throughout a difficult life of pain and suffering. While he will be sorely missed, we rejoice at his final release from the purgatory on earth that was his lot. Heaven has to be a brighter place because of him, and on Earth, ours a sadder lot. From his natural father, to reflect on God's words: "This is my son, of whom I am most proud."

Always and forever a part of us...his father and mother, Bob and Jane Weeber; his alter ego, best friend and twin brother, Nicky; sisters Wanda and Mary, Uncle Armin and Niece Katie, and "Max" the cat, also died April 3, 1993. May God receive Bobby and hold him dear for us.

A memorial service was held at Summerville Presbyterian Church April 6, 1993

Contents

Preface

As a young girl growing up in rural North Carolina, my wife's plans, dreams, and hopes were the same as countless other young girls of her time…to get married, have children, but above all, to want and expect them to be healthy and normal. The very thought that they would be less than perfect was abhorrent to her. The possibility that she could wind up having not just one, but two babies at a time, terribly afflicted, never entered her thinking—yet, that is exactly what happened.

We married during war time and both of us were young. Shortly after I completed my World War II service, we had our first child. Our daughter, who, although sickly, did not manifest any serious disorder. After a thirteen-year interval, a second daughter was born. Outside of developing a cataract in one eye at the age of two and a half, she was healthy and normal.

In July of 1962, identical twin sons were born, during a difficult delivery. I was forty four—Jane was forty. Almost half a year later, a determined member of our pediatric team finally put the pieces of the puzzle together. The positive diagnosis: NEURO-FIBROMA-TOSIS, a then totally obscure disease about which almost nothing was known even by professionals whose business was to know and understand such things. It would explain why the twins acted as if they were possessed by the devil himself. Their affliction was congenital, a product of a mutation of the genes, characterized by tumors (usually benign, but potentially cancerous) that can disfigure, disable, and/or kill. Throw in predictions of mental retardation, plus the probability of a relatively early death—age twenty one or sooner—and we found ourselves confronted with a grim outlook.

Thus began, in earnest, the saga of "GOD'S CAREGIVERS—A Journey of Faith". At this juncture, there was nowhere else to turn to but Faith. And thirty-nine years later, Faith is still the main ingredient that keeps things going.

From the onset, we were soldiers in charge of battles for our mutual survival, conducted on multiple fronts simultaneously.

What we faced was a lack of understanding from more than one direction. From professionals who should have known better; educators, many of whom needed educating themselves and attitudes; even our own family members (that can best be described as denial) to society in general, many members of which equated the twins' physical problems with presumed retardation.

Struggles for benefits; problems with home health care agencies and aides; dealings with neurosurgeons, all of whom were at the top of their profession, but some temperamentally difficult; hospitals, both general and rehab, along with nursing homes, tested out mettle and resolve. Courageous sums up how the boys dealt with their lives.

Our immediate family consisted of my wife Jane, twins and me. Jane and I were the primary caregivers and the only family members who have ever been involved in caring for our identical twin sons, Bobby and Nicky, from the time they entered the public school system to the present. I jokingly explain that Jane and I have over one hundred sixty years of experience between us, since I am eighty three and Jane was seventy seven. Believe us, there have been many times when we needed to call on every one of those one hundred sixty years to handle situations involving one or more of our four children!

Nicholas David Weeber (Nicky) and Robert Vincent Weeber (Bobby) were born July 12, 1962, with extremely severe cases of Neuro-Fibroma-Tosis,about which little was known at the time. One of Bobby's countless tumors became cancerous, and since it was attached to his spinal cord, no surgery was possible. He passed away April 3rd,

1993. Nicky, the surviving twin, was being maintained at home by us, with the assistance of home health care aides.

Both boys graduated from a Special Education program in the York Suburban school district in York County, Pennsylvania. They were classed as "learning disabled" to be eligible for acceptance.

The two daughters are now living in nearby states. Wanda Jane, our first born daughter has retired from her job as a high school teacher in Duval County (Jacksonville), Florida school system. Her husband, Warren Hogan, is an officer in the Duval County Sheriff's Department. They have one daughter, Katie, who graduated from college at Florida State University in Tallahassee, Florida.

Mary Kathryn Bell is a Major Accounts Representative for BellSouth Yellow Pages and lives in Suwanee, Georgia with her husband John and son, Joshua Taylor.

Both daughters graduated from college with honors. They were each awarded honor scholarships.

While both Wanda and Mary—and their children—have had numerous physical health problems, ranging from severe to mild, neither daughter nor their children have shown any signs of neuro-fibroma-tosis, for which we are all grateful. Because of their work and family obligations, plus their distance from us, neither daughter can give us any respite from our caregiver duties. They lack the physical strength required to handle transfers of Nicky. Five or six of these are necessary each and every day and with few exceptions, two persons are needed to do them.

My brother, Armin Weeber was eighty-four years old and could not handle Nicky by himself. Although, in 1990, when Bobby was at Duke Medical Center for five weeks, following his last spinal cord decompression surgery, Armin watched out for Nicky at home here in Summerville, while we made five weekly round trips to Duke Hospital to see Bobby and comfort him during his recovery. He could walk then with a walker. Armin's help was really appreciated.

After four major operations to remove tumors (a procedure known as decompressing the spinal cord), a usually benign tumor attached to the spinal cord became cancerous and Bobby passed away at age thirty-one, beating the premature death prediction by ten years. Nicky, the surviving twin, now lives in a group home in South Carolina as a quadriplegic. He has overcome almost all of the manifestations of retardation and/or learning disability and as did his brother, earned the respect of his ministers and the entertainment figures that he contacts by phone and mail.

For over thirty-nine years, it has been—and is to this day—an ongoing case of abiding love and care tendered by us as their parents and driven by a combination of love, faith, obligation, and necessity.

Along the way, those both in and out of churches who were not afraid to care, helped ease the trauma of a succession of crises that involved neurosurgeons and hospitals, rehab centers, nursing homes, insurance companies, Medicaid, Medicare, SSI, The South Carolina Department of Disabilities and Special Needs (their predecessor, The South Carolina Department of Mental Retardation), a seemingly endless parade of half a dozen home health care agencies and over two hundred home health care aides, The South Carolina Department of Social Services and South Carolina Community Long Term Care were also among the entities involved.

"You Are Heroes to Me....
Because You're Doing God's Work"

When we received our then minister's letter containing the above words, my wife and I were startled. Coming from a person we looked up to as a compelling speaker, highly intelligent, a dedicated servant of God, and a true friend, we were flattered. But we wondered.

We certainly never set out to be heroes, and we're still not certain that we are worthy of the many accolades that have come our way. We acted as caregivers out of love for both boys, with compassion for their plight as the primary motivation. There is, along with this love, a deep sense of obligation. They didn't ask to come into this world. None of us wanted them to be so horribly stricken with such a major disease as neuro-fibroma-tosis (nerve tumors).

But, from their birth on, we accepted the challenge. We had no choice. We have been told many times by many persons what a great job we are doing. Comments range from "I don't see how you both do it, at your ages, and keep doing it, without letting it destroy you", to "As bad as it must be for Bobby and Nicky, how lucky they are to have you two to give them the loving care that you do".

The lady typesetter who set type for the "In Memoriam" eulogy about Bobby as he was in his final earthly days, and who was aware of his life and death because of that, asked me, "How in the world could you and your wife handle the agony of Bobby's terminal illness and death"?

My answer was that it was the most difficult thing that any parent could ever be called upon to go through…to confirm to your son that, unless divine intervention ensued, or a medical miracle, he was destined to leave us, and pass on to a kinder, gentler existence. His breathing became more labored and difficult from the tremendous tumor that was slowly crushing him and his death appeared imminent. It was agonizing for Nicky to witness the life literally being squeezed out of Bobby and with a sense of disbelief he observed the unfolding tragedy.

I remember what happened next as if it were yesterday. Bobby, Nicky and I were in Bobby's room, where he and Nicky spent their days. The answer to my dilemma about how and when to tell Bobby that his condition had been ruled terminal, was about to be solved in a most unexpected manner.

Nicky began reading out loud, a letter that he had written earlier that day. It was addressed to a female soap opera TV star with which both boys had often corresponded. In it, he mentioned that Bobby was terminal and never hesitated to read it, not realizing that Bobby himself had not been told. It started out: "Dear Star: Hello from Summerville,

South Carolina! My back is hurting me today. Our cat, Max is not well. We plan to take him to the vet today. The weather here has been chilly and rainy and more is expected. Bobby has a growth on his side and his doctor says that he is terminal. Write when you can". Love, Nicky.

When the word "terminal" came out, there was an anguished cry of protest from Bobby. I, in turn, felt as if a dagger had been plunged into my heart. I had wanted to tell Bobby privately, with Jane also present, but Nicky had beaten us to it. Of course, it had to come out sooner or later, but this wasn't the way I had planned it. In reality, no good way existed.

In the stress of the moment, I regret that I reprimanded Nicky severely, yelling at him "You never should have read that letter out loud in front of Bobby", and asked him to leave the room. Nicky replied (as close to tears as he and Bobby would ever get), "Daddy, I didn't know that Bobby didn't know".

Bobby's face was ashen, as if all the color had been drained out of it, and he was visibly agitated, shaking like a leaf. My heart went out to him. I wanted to ease the terror that he was experiencing, but what to say? Bobby turned to me and implored me to tell Nicky that he must be mistaken—that I'm not terminal. There was nothing that I could think of to make this nightmarish situation any better. But as traumatic as it was going to be on Bobby, the truth had to be revealed.

"Bobby", I assured him as I put my arms around him, "I'm afraid that Nicky has it right. Without divine intervention or a medical miracle, your condition has been declared terminal by your neurosurgeon." I saw the disbelief in his eyes and had to fight back the tears myself.

Bobby cried out, his voice choked up. "This is terrible—it means that I won't be around any more. What did I do to deserve this? I've tried to be a good son". I assured him that he had indeed been a good son; not only a good son, but one of the finest sons that any parents could possibly have hoped for. I told him that God was not punishing him, but on the contrary, was moving to end the cruel and relentless pain he had been suffering for the past many weeks and years.

Trying to console Bobby, I told him, "You can't continue to live in agony, with the tumor crushing you and getting larger. There has to be something better in store for you, where you can exist free of pain and live in peace. We'll always love you, you'll always be a part of our family and we'll miss you, for all the days of our lives".

I felt that my words to him, spoken with all the conviction that I could muster, had a reassuring effect on Bobby. He appeared to have recovered from his upset over the unintentional revelation of his terminal illness, and from then on, even more than could be expected, he was accepting of his fate, and began preparing for it.

Like the champion that he was, there was no whimpering or hysterics. On his final day, he asked Jane and I to pray out loud, not just with him, but for him. We stood on either side of his hospital bed, each of us holding one of his hands. I am positive that I saw a wisp of what appeared to be white threads ascend over him—his soul rising.

I suggested that Bobby forgive the legions of persons who had sneered at him, made fun of him, ridiculed him and otherwise made his life miserable. In effect, to accept the fact that they didn't know any better. Pity them, be sorry for them, forgive them, but don't hate them. He agreed.

He wanted to give us the few dollars that he had in his wallet. I thanked him, but suggested that he give it to his brother, to which he readily consented.

When the same minister who wrote us that we were his heroes delivered Bobby's eulogy at his Memorial Service, he mentioned that he had learned the true meaning of grace from both Bobby and Nicky.

This tribute, to such excellent character as the boys exhibited is one of the many factors that prompts this account of their lives and our experiences in caring for them. It also gives them some measure of credit for making such a valiant attempt to overcome the condition of having intelligent minds imprisoned in bodies that refused to cooperate, and to serve as an inspiration to others.

We hope that this chronicle will serve to inspire some of the army of caregivers who may find themselves in similar circumstances. If it helps to fortify your sense of obligation, of duty, concern and compassion, and last, but not least, of genuine love, then it will have been worth the effort and pain in recalling the past events, dealing with the current reality, and facing the future with faith in God to continue His support for our commitment.

WHY "GOD'S CAREGIVERS"?

We wish to make it abundantly clear that the selection of "God's Caregivers" as a title of this work is based entirely on the assessment of what we are doing by several members of the clergy, along with comments by many others, from all walks of life. It is not a self-appointed label that we have placed upon ourselves, but we are proud to be counted among that number.

There is no questions but that anyone and everyone who acts in a loving, faithful and conscientious manner to give care to another human being, is doing "God's work" and is therefore a member of the legions who belong to this group. None are uniquely greater or more blessed than any others who also provide love and abiding care, nor do genuine caregivers seek material rewards or praise for what they do.

CHAPTER ONE

Our Extended Family

From the very first, beginning with the boys' birth in 1962, and continuing to this very day, our family members have been involved in the twins' lives, to varying degrees. Most are mentioned in the account that follows. Some took part briefly, a few for a longer time. We acknowledge, with gratitude, their participation, however much or little it may have been.

Both my mother, Harriet Weeber and Jane's mother, Ida Adcock, were very fond of the twins. For a brief period before the boys' birth in July of 1962, my mother lived with us. We desperately needed more room, and ordered construction to start on a larger house. Included was a "mother-in-law wing", plus three other bedrooms. Mrs. Adcock contributed to the cost and came to live with us until she passed on in 1969.

After supper, almost every night, grandmother Adcock waited for the boys to get into their pajamas and come to her bedroom, where she read to them from books for children. Often we heard them laughing their heads off. Once in a while, they would act rowdy and misbehave, whereupon grandmother would put down the book, close up shop, and send them packing back to our side of the house. She continued reading to them right up to her death. The boys were too young to have many memories of her, but she loved them dearly.

My mother and Jane did not get along. She lived with us on and off; she finally left for good and eventually got a home of her own, provided by my brother, Armin. My mother always remembered the boys at

Easter, their birthdays, and Christmas, although her resources were limited. She passed away in 1983, at the age of ninety-three.

Wanda, our first child, was born June 30, 1946, in the vanguard of what later came to be known as "Baby Boomers". When the boys were born in 1962, Wanda was thirteen. A couple of years later, she was off to college for four years and in 1970, she married. By then, the boys were eight and just entering into the special-education program offered by the public school system.

In effect, Wanda did not grow up with Bobby and Nicky. She missed being personally involved or aware first hand of the trials and tribulations their very existence created. As a result, there was not the closeness that developed between the boys and Mary, our second child. She was eleven when we all moved to York, PA in order for me to pursue a career advancement. When we arrived in York, both Mary and the boys were enrolled in the same elementary school for a brief period of time.

When Wanda was very little, she and I were very close—Daddy's little girl. Even though now married, I know that she missed both Jane and me after we left Jacksonville, Florida, although in the eighteen years we were in York, there were frequent visits back and forth.

After Bobby passed on, Wanda moved closer to Nicky. Also, she wrote a genuinely touching poem, entitled "My Brother Bobby". We still exchange visits and the "Baby Boomer" just retired from her job as a high school teacher. Her husband, Warren Hogan, is a retired police officer in the Duval County, Florida Sheriff's Department. A computer enthusiast , Warren would be very helpful to Nicky if he lived closer to us. Now that Nicky has WEB TV, he is excited by the opportunity to send and receive E-Mail. Nicky received a very nice E-Mail message from his Jacksonville brother-in-law and we're hoping that Warren's computer and Nicky's WEB TV can bridge the miles.

Mary was pregnant with Joshua when Bobby passed away April 3, 1993. She came to the viewing and for the Memorial Service at our church and took his death very hard. Mary was extremely close to both boys. She was careful to think of things for them all of their holidays and birthdays she generously remembered. Even more appreciated were frequent phone calls to see how they were doing, and to encourage them. When we had a point to get across to Bobby and Nicky, which they either were resisting, or we felt they would resist, we would enlist Mary's aid and she was usually very effective in persuading them. They listened to her.

She has continued with Nicky, perhaps with even a more visible concern for his welfare. Despite her own sizeable responsibilities as a top producer for the Atlanta area BellSouth Yellow Pages, plus parenting Joshua, she stays on top of Nicky's situation and its impact on Jane and me. Mary's husband, John Bell, takes enormous amounts of time to talk to Nicky, listening to what he has to say and making a genuine effort to share his expertise on whatever subject with which Nicky needs help. John and Mary decided that WEB TV would be "just what the doctor ordered" for Nicky and they have very generously provided the necessary equipment. Not only that, John has devoted many hours tutoring Nicky and constantly helps Nicky by phone through some puzzling happenings on the WEB. Several friends previewed advance copies of "GOD'S CAREGIVERS" and asked, "Where were Jane and Nicky in your story"? A good question. Because you're not going to read about Jane a great deal. The same is true of Nicky, although to a lesser degree.

Nicky's reluctance to be featured in this account, any more than necessary, is due to one fundamental reason: he finds it too painful. He misses Bobby terribly. As identical twins, they were mirror images of each other. When Bobby passed on, he literally took part of Nicky with him. Studies of identical twins indicate that they tend to weaken one another because they are very close and depend on each other to the exclusion of others in the family circle. Therefore, since Bobby's passing, I see Nicky strengthened in many areas, such as assertiveness—he no longer has Bobby to turn to and has had to develop his own personality to a greater degree than he otherwise would have.

There are some small samples of Nicky's writing in the Appendix. I've pleaded with him to write about the many times that he and Bobby talked and planned together. I felt that this would open up thoughts and ideas he and Bobby shared of which even I am probably unaware. But the answer remains the same—"too painful", and since that is the case, I cannot force the issue.

On a recent Thanksgiving Day, Jane and I remarked that "Macy's" traditional parade looked very spectacular on TV and reminded Nicky that it should be worth his tuning in, especially since he sees a lot of TV and is an excellent judge and critic. He was adamant that he did not intend to watch it. Finally I asked why. His answer came in an emotional voice: "Because Bobby and I used to watch it together". That kind of painful memory could generate anger on Nicky's part against the circumstances that took Bobby from him, and could very well some day take Nicky himself away from us.

Jane's response was a great deal more complicated. She has consistently been there for the boys and me throughout this long ordeal, applying her common sense and a mother's love to handle difficult events on an almost daily basis.

Like Nicky, Jane would tell you that many of the problems we've faced are too painful to relive. If there were no current matters to deal with, reliving the past would be a lot easier, but such is not the case, and never will be.

Jane was an honestly self-effacing type of person. If others want to say that she's some kind of "Steel Magnolia", that's okay, but you'll never hear her proclaim that kind of description of herself. On the other hand, she has handled many trying situations with resolve and made countless decisions that are effective and fit the circumstances well.

Jane would be the first to admit that, give a choice, she would much rather be doing what many retirees are free to do—such as extended visits with friends and relatives, and now and then, a trip to a new area.

Perhaps more time for gardening or reading, or the option not to have to do anything. But no such choice is available.

It has fallen to me to take the lead in almost every phase of our involvement in caring for the boys. The long list includes (but is not limited to): getting them the best medical care possible, from pediatricians to neurosurgeons to family doctors; fighting to obtain benefits from Medicare, Medicaid, Social Security disability; the Departments of Social Services in both York County, PA and Dorchester County, SC; The South Carolina Department of Disabilities and Special Needs and their predecessor, The South Carolina Department of Mental Retardation; The York Guidance Clinic; The York-Adams Mental Health-Mental Retardation Agency; the public school systems in Duval County, FL and York County, PA and The Lincoln Intermediate Unit in New Oxford, PA for their special education needs.

To these can be added a host of medical equipment providers, countless pharmacies for the boys' prescription needs, plus physical therapists, dentists, optometrists and a number of medical specialists. At least half a dozen general hospitals in three states; a nursing home, and a rehab hospital along with a rehab unit in a general hospital, round out the list.

Jane's counsel, suggestions and input on all of the areas mentioned has been invaluable. In many instances, following her assessments has often resulted in better outcomes than if my conclusions had been followed.

The one sector that Jane has been almost one hundred percent in charge of is home health care agencies and the home health care aides that come. Well over two hundred aides have been sent to us since we started in 1991 and we are currently having staffing problems with agency number six.

The lack of staffing to fill the time slots scheduled for Nicky's program, plus the questionable quality of many of the aides, has been the source of much frustration and many arguments between both Jane and me and between her and the agency.

CHAPTER TWO

Your Sons Are Retarded—
And You'll Have to Learn to Live With It!

We had been having a difficult time with the newborn twins ever since their birth. They were extremely hyperactive, restless, and irritable. They had us up all night long, crying, twisting and tossing. No sleep pattern was emerging...pacifiers no longer pacified (even after we repeatedly dipped them in a mixture of rum and honey).

We knew that something was radically wrong—and the team of well-experienced pediatricians was aware of it, but no one seemed able to get the handle on it. This added large amounts of fear and frustration to the situation and we were getting desperate for some kind of reason for their obvious discomfort—a reason we hoped would lead to steps that could be taken to improve things—for the boys' sake and ours.

When the lead doctor told me on the phone, "Your sons are retarded and you'll have to learn to live with it", my first reaction was anger. The conclusion was wrong and in fact just couldn't be. No indication appeared in either of our family trees of anything approaching retardation. In fact, the reverse was true—above average and even superior intelligence on both sides.

The "conclusion" was voiced coldly. I was too stunned to question the findings, or to ask on what evidence the doctor had formed his opinion. It was, as it turned out, just his opinion, unsupported, at this point, by any scientific research or study. The boys were now about three months old.

Jane might have been more inclined to go along with the retardation diagnosis than I was. She was to tell me, several years down the line, that, when they brought the twins to her hospital bed to see and to hold, she felt instinctively that "something" was not quite right about them. Call if a mother's gut feeling, but she concluded that trouble loomed ahead, hoping that events would prove her fears to be unfounded.

Dr. Roberts, who had assumed the lead in the twins' case at his pediatric practice, suggested that we take the boys to specialists in Gainesville, Florida.

The J. Hillis Miller Medical Center at The University of Florida, in Gainesville, Florida, was establishing a reputation for handling problem cases, finding reasons and reaching conclusions that other medical facilities had trouble reaching. To be back where I had been a student as a freshman in 1936, a good quarter of a century previous, felt strange.

We had to leave the twins for four days and three nights. We were told that they would be doing liver tests; a possible liver malfunction might be the answer to the puzzle. I especially remember observing them tied down to their hospital beds with strips of gauze. They looked so tiny and helpless, straining to break the bonds that held them and set themselves free. But the answer was not found there and we returned home to Jacksonville, Florida, discouraged at the lack of positive results. The twins were about four months old at this point.

Unbeknownst to us, Dr. Roberts had continued to search for the diagnosis. Though a Board Certified Pediatrician, his bedside manner was that of a "country" doctor. Even though he had not attended a prestigious Medical School, such as Duke University or Harvard, he did research and studied what was available at that time. A "hunch" he termed it later.

Upon our return from J. Hillis Miller Medical Center in Gainesville, Dr. Roberts called Jane and me into his office and told us that he was now able to tell us, with certainty, exactly what the twins' diagnosis was. A congenital condition called neuro-fibroma-tosis, a serious disease that we had never heard of (and soon were to find out, many health professionals also had little or no knowledge of).

In medical school, Dr. Roberts had read about the work of a German, Dr. Freidrich von Recklinghausen, who had, in 1882, delineated a genetic disorder that caused tumors and could be recognized early on by a number of characteristics. One was the presence of light brown spots on the skin, known as "café-au-lait". Both boys had these markings in several areas on their skin—Bobby had twenty-two, Nicky, twelve.

He requested that we permit him and one of his partners, to present the boys, in person, together with their findings and diagnosis, to a panel of physicians and surgeons. This took place at St. Vincent's Hospital in Jacksonville, Florida. The boys were about seven months old and had been hospitalized for a week. Their presentation, with the twins in a single wheelchair, made it possible for the panel of doctors to observe the boys—especially the skin color markings. Other physical indicators were also pointed out. Their findings of neuro-fibroma-tosis were confirmed.

We had been told that the condition of NF was a serious disease and that for either twin to live beyond age twenty-one would be a minor miracle. Learning disabilities would be a prevalent as well.

Two distinct battles for their welfare now began. One was the educational situation, the other coping with the effects of NF, neurosurgeons calling it two of the most severe cases they were aware of.

WHAT WE LEARNED ABOUT OUR DOCTOR'S DIAGNOSIS OF RETARDATION, NEURO-FIBROMA-TOSIS AND EARLY DEATH FOR OUR SONS

While our doctors used their best judgment, based on what was known at the time, not all of their predictions have come to pass.

While Bobby did pass away much too early, both boys lived well beyond age 21, and Nicky is now 39.

As for retardation, the word itself is frightening to most people…but it really means "slow", which can be mild to severe.

Early automobiles had a lever on or near the steering wheel marked "Retard" and that helped slow the vehicle down. Both boys developed excellent vocabularies, as well as effective verbal and written skills.

NF is still with us and as yet there is no cure. We pray that day will come soon.

CHAPTER THREE

The Medical Merry-Go-Round
(Or, Getting Your Doctor's Attention)

In 1968, when Bobby was six years old, he was taken to Hope Haven Hospital in Jacksonville, Florida, to have a herniated navel repaired. A routine chest X-ray done there revealed the existence of an egg-sized tumor. Jane and I waited outside in the hospital courtyard, looking up at the large window area on the second floor, where the surgeons were operating. Afterwards, Jane saw the tumor in a jar in his hospital room and I saw a hospital orderly going down a hall with the jar in his hand. The tumor proved to be benign.

Sometime in 1972, two years after arriving in York, Pennsylvania, we took the boys to John Hopkins Medical University in Baltimore, Maryland to be examined by the Chief Neurosurgeon. He took one look at them and made an instant evaluation: neuro-fibroma-tosis—learning disability!

In 1977-78, Nicky and Bobby, at ages fifteen-sixteen, were seen in the Outpatient Clinic at Elizabethtown Hospital for Children and Youth, in Elizabethtown, Pennsylvania, for possible scoliosis correction. In 1978, after five or six months of Clinic visits (one hundred-mile round trips to and from Elizabethtown back to York), a spinal fusion was done on Bobby at Hershey Medical Center in Hershey, Pennsylvania. Dr. Edward Schwenkert, Hospital Director at Elizabethtown, operated. Bobby was placed in a heavy body cast and returned to Elizabethtown Children's Hospital for rehabilitation. The entire procedure took two months.

We made frequent visits to see Bobby and would buy him his favorite foods—hamburgers and fries—from a local restaurant. Bobby formed a close attachment to his nurse, Kathryn Beck. They entered into a correspondence that has lasted over twenty years, exchanging about two letters a month. The operation didn't achieve the desired results but Bobby stood taller and much straighter for several months.

As the boys began to grow and develop, so did their tumors. Those on the skin surface could be removed with relative ease by a plastic surgeon. These operations were done in the doctor's office, with local anesthesia. Because Bobby's case was more severe than Nicky's, he had more tumors that needed removing. The general rule was not to bother the tumors until they either became painful or showed signs of abscessing.

As the boys' condition gradually worsened, the tumors were growing internally, compressing the spinal cord, shutting down the nervous system, and creating sharp, stabbing pains. Their plastic surgeon told me about the chief neurosurgeon at Children's Hospital in Philadelphia, Dr. Luis Schute.

We contacted Dr. Schute's office and a three month effort of phone calls and letters began, pleading for an appointment for Bobby. Nothing was forthcoming. Bobby was now barely able to move with a walker. Finally, we obtained an appointment for both boys to be seen by Dr. Schute. After he saw Bobby and Nicky, he remarked to Jane, "Yes, Bobby needs help".

Dr. Schute ordered an MRI (Magnetic Resonance Imaging) test to be done on both boys. These produce a high-resolution picture (aided by dye injected in the patient), showing in more detail than a CAT scan could, the internal location and size of the tumors and their relative location to the spinal cord. He requested that these tests be done at The University of Pennsylvania Medical Center, which was adjacent to Children's Hospital.

Another waiting period commenced, with no response from Dr. Schute. Bobby's condition continued to deteriorate. In desperation, I went back to his plastic surgeon, Dr. Davis and asked, "Will you please intervene on Bobby's behalf, call Dr. Schute, find out, will he operate on Bobby or not? We need to know, since there is no one in York who will take his case". Dr. Davis said he would see what he could do.

Why the uncertainty, why the long delay in coming to a decision? At the time, we had no idea. In retrospect, a number of factors appeared at work. Neurosurgeons such as Dr. Schute are at the top of a very demanding profession. They enjoy international reputations and their patients come to them from all over the world (the boys would later see three more neurosurgeons of comparable stature). They can be selective. They also would seem to prefer that the patient urgently request their services and to ask them very strongly for their help. This tends to avoid the appearance of "pushing" for an operation. Further, the boys were now twenty-two years old, well beyond the upper age limit for children to be admitted to Children's Hospital. And they doubtlessly didn't want to operate on patients whom they are certain they cannot help, as became the case later with Bobby and Nicky.

Finally, Dr. Schute made the decision to operate. We took Bobby to Children's Hospital for pre-operative testing and returned to York to care for Nicky. Dr. Schute said that he would personally operate and promised to call us immediately after the operation. He said that they would use laser, ultra sound dissection, and surgical knives to remove the tumors.

The operations started around 7 a.m. Children's Hospital is a teaching institution, so Dr. Schute had his senior assistants with him, as well as student neurosurgeons, some doing their residency and others in varying stages of knowledge, experience and medical education.

The operation continued for nine hours. We waited anxiously and prayed earnestly. Around supper time, Dr. Schute called. Bobby was in intensive care and recovery, in stable condition. Two medium to large size tumors had been removed (although some vestiges of each still remained). He termed the operation a success. We talked to Bobby on the phone the next morning and the following day we took Nicky and journeyed to Philadelphia to see Bobby. He could now wiggle his toes, an improvement.

He was to stay in the hospital for ten days, during which they commenced physical therapy to see if he was able to stand and/or walk. We decided that he needed to go directly from the hospital, on discharge, to York Rehabilitation Hospital in York, Pennsylvania. This was a new, state-of-the-art rehab facility, run by a doctor who was himself wheelchair bound.

But after a few days there, Bobby was vomiting so badly that he couldn't eat. No one seemed able to get the handle on it.

After a few more days, I got Dr. Schute on the phone, outlining to him what I felt was a desperate situation. To my surprise, he said, "We have nothing further to offer Bobby here", and terminated the conversation. My heart was in my mouth, my thoughts full of fear and confusion. What do we do now?

It was Friday. I gathered my courage together and called back to Children's Hospital. I honestly don't know—years later—who I talked to. I said that we would be bringing Bobby back on Saturday, win, lose, or draw. We knew that at least a resident neurosurgeon would be on duty. Sure enough, upon our arrival, we were directed to Dr. Bell, who saw Bobby in the emergency room, after only a short wait.

The fact that we now had someone to turn to who would try to find the problem, reassured us that we had done the right thing. After a brief discussion, Dr. Bell performed a spinal tap. His diagnosis was right on—Bobby had been losing spinal fluid, which disrupted his system and made him ill. A shunt was necessary to relieve the condition. We thanked Dr. Bell profusely and Bobby stayed behind as we once again returned to our home in York, Pennsylvania.

On the following Monday, Dr. Bruce, who was a senior associate with Dr. Schute, operated on Bobby and installed a shunt in his abdomen.

Bobby stayed in the hospital for a few more days, following which we again came back to Philadelphia to return him to York Rehab Hospital.

But there the vomiting continued unabated. After calling Philadelphia, we were told to bring Bobby back. We did, and this time a connector shunt was installed, running from the base of his skull downward, connecting with the shunt already in place in his abdomen. This finally stopped the fluid from leaking. After a short discussion, we opted to bring him directly home.

During this initial ordeal, Bobby made many friends. Relatives of fellow patients, hospital staffers, and a multitude of doctors, admired his demeanor and long before the movie *Grace Under Fire* was ever thought of, he surely was the personification of that. He deserved the compliments. Sure, he had some complaints when things got out of hand, but for the most part, he took the knocks without whimpering. A class act, if ever there was one.

In late 1984, as Bobby was in recovery, Nicky also became paralyzed from the hips down, unable to stand or walk. Once again, we called Children's Hospital. Nicky was admitted December 9th for evaluation and tests and was discharged December 11th. Nicky certainly didn't want to spend Christmas Day in any hospital unless absolutely necessary. And that went for the doctors and nurses too, I'm sure.

On January 13, 1985, we took Nicky back to Philadelphia and he was again admitted. Because his case was not as severe as Bobby's and the surgeons had recent experience with his identical twin brother, the operation took six hours instead of nine. As before, we returned to York, were notified by phone, and were there the next day to comfort Nicky as best we could.

When Bobby had his operation, they put an inner-city street-guy type in the same room with him. He harassed Bobby repeatedly, threw his eyeglasses in the trash (we were never able to find them), bolted the door to their room and refused to open it, and threatened to kill Bobby.

Complaints to the charge nurse were futile. The hospital obviously felt that its hands were tied.

As a result, before Nicky was admitted, I went to the Assistant Hospital Administrator, explained how Bobby was mistreated and insisted that Nicky be placed in a safer section of the hospital. They put him in a separate room, in the pediatric ward on another floor, with no teen-age hoodlums. We brought Nicky home after about a week of physical therapy and he too walked again.

In 1987, three years after his operation at Children's Hospital of Philadelphia, Bobby was again experiencing spinal compression, barely able to get around with a cane. This new development would prove, for Bobby, to be part of a series of paralysis, surgery to decompress the spinal cord, and recovery—in almost even three-year cycles!

Since Hershey was half as far as Philadelphia from where we lived, and because they had medical records already on file from the boys' previous evaluation there in 1982, we decided that we would place him in their hands. Both hospitals were state-of-the-art, but the Hershey complex was newer, and growing. Plus, the setting was right in the middle of the famous "Pennsylvania Dutch" farmland country, as opposed to the grim surroundings in urban Pennsylvania. Bobby's Hershey records were updated and certain records and scans were obtained from Children's Hospital (after considerable effort).

Just before Thanksgiving, Bobby was operated on by Dr. Lehman, the Chief Neurosurgeon, and his "team". As before, we were at home with Nicky and got the call from Dr. Lehman that the operation had been completed (another nine-hour time frame) with no complications. Bobby was in intensive care and could be seen the following day. The surgeons had removed most of the tumors that Dr. Lehman had judged to be the cause of his leg paralysis.

Once again, we began the almost daily commute to visit Bobby. Jane did not come every time, as she had to work at her job as supervisor of policy typing at Continental Insurance Company's regional office in

York. I brought Nicky along and since Bobby wouldn't eat the hospital food, I wound up getting both boys hamburgers or chicken legs and french fries for lunch.

After a week, during which Thanksgiving came and went, Bobby was transferred back to Elizabethtown Hospital, which had now become a full-fledged division of Hershey Medical Center, operating as a rehabilitation center.

This time, Bobby was placed in the spinal cord injury section. Almost all the patients were youthful accident victims, some becoming instant paraplegics or quadriplegics.

Bobby complained to me that he couldn't understand why psychiatrists kept coming by and asking him if he were contemplating suicide. Of course, he told them no. But for many young patients in that ward, their current condition, along with their bleak futures had them thinking such thoughts and the rehab hospital was trying to counsel them not to take that step.

A male aide assigned to Bobby had a sinister-looking face accentuated by his heavy, black beard and dark complexion. After a few days, Bobby told me that the guy was, as they say nowadays, "talking trash". His remarks and comments were not designed to improve anyone's morale, especially these patients in that ward. They certainly didn't need someone taking his life's problems out. I finally began making discreet inquiries about what was ailing him, prior to going to the Rehab Director, to voice a complaint. Before I was able to do that, I was told that the aide had submitted his resignation and was working his final days as an employee. Thank God! If, when they hired him, they were trying to find the one person who could do the most damage to a patient's morale and the hospital's recovery efforts, they couldn't have made a better choice!

After about a month of physical therapy, Bobby was discharged. Two good things came out of it all. Kathryn Beck, the nurse that Bobby had bonded with in 1978, when he had his spinal fusion, came by several times to visit with him and also talked to him on the phone.

Also, because they were not sure how well he would be able to get around and because they were made aware that our family was planning a move completely out of the Pennsylvania area, they decided that he should have a manual wheelchair.

Because of a misunderstanding, we mistakenly failed to notify our private health insurer *before* the operation was performed. As a result of this, payment of our claim was reduced drastically, leaving us with a potential liability of about four thousand dollars. Fortunately, we were able to show that this was a procedural error caused, in large part, by misinformation furnished to us by Jane's employer at their home office in New York City. Full payment of the claim was authorized. Just another day at the office!

Bobby came back from the operation and could walk with a cane— for a while.

When we arrived in the "Low Country" of South Carolina in April 1988, we immediately registered both boys with the neurosurgical department of The Medical University of South Carolina. MUSC is another teaching institution and the chief neurosurgeon, Dr. Phanor Perot, Jr., is another top-notch neurosurgeon with an international reputation. When Dr. Lehman, at Hershey Medical Center, found out that we were coming to the Charleston, South Carolina area, he urged us to contact Dr. Perot and assured us that the boys would receive excellent care in his hands.

We were initially assigned an associate professor in the neurosurgical department, Dr. Alfred Nelson, Jr. We arranged for the boys to have routine checks twice a year and they had MRI's done at a MUSC facility. In a few years, Dr. Nelson moved to Greenville, South Carolina and Dr. Perot himself took over the boys' care.

In 1990, following the three-year cycle of operation, recovery and paralysis, Bobby was again having great difficulty in walking from one end of our house to the other. He had slowly gone from a cane to a walker and now that wasn't enough, so we resorted to the wheelchair that the Elizabethtown Rehab Center had so thoughtfully ordered.

Bobby again, needed help, and we approached Dr. Perot. Current MRI scans were made, and based on these, plus his knowledge of the case, Dr. Perot told us he could not and would not operate.

Frustrated, we had to turn elsewhere, since MUSC neurosurgery was "the only game in town". Mayo Clinic had a facility in Jacksonville, Florida. We had lived there from 1940 to 1970 and had family there. As a matter of fact, all four of our children were born in Jacksonville, Florida. Despite Mayo Clinic's prestigious reputation, their neuro-surgery department apparently depended upon some kind of closed-circuit communication with their main headquarters in Minneapolis. For that reason, we ruled it out.

Dr. Perot gave us the name of Dr. Robert Wilkins, chief neurosur-geon at Duke Medical Center, Duke University, Durham, North Carolina. Dr. Wilkins was yet another renowned neurosurgeon, with a sterling reputation, in a teaching institution environment. I mention "teaching institution" because we soon found out that unless a neuro-surgeon was in an institution where training and development of future neurosurgeons was ongoing, the depth of experience and facilities sim-ply were not sufficient to handle the severity of the twin's condition.

I contacted his office by phone, working at first through his secre-taries. They were truly outstanding and seemed to clearly understand and be concerned about out predicament. I told them that Dr. Perot felt that he could not operate, fearing he might to more harm than good. More than once, to prove his point and justify his decision not to oper-ate on either boy, he would ask me to come to an area in his department where x-rays, CAT scans, and MRI results were displayed against a lighted background. They clearly showed countless sizeable tumors, close to or attached to the spinal cord—at every level of both the cervi-cal and thoracic spine. He would say, "Which ones do I remove? I simply cannot be sure". He would turn to me for answer, knowing that, least of all, did I have an answer to the question.

I asked for an appointment with Dr. Wilkins *for myself,* to avoid Bobby's having to make a grueling five hundred fifty mile round trip if no hope existed for him at all, intending to plead his case with Dr. Wilkins. I would bring all the MRI scans with me (and I had a stack of them), plus all of the written reports I had on Bobby from Children's Hospital, Hershey Medical Center, and MUSC. Finally, Dr. Wilkins agreed that I could do this.

I was apprehensive, feeling that what might be our son's last chance rested on how convincing I could be, and how it would be received by the doctor.

I was ushered into a small patient's waiting room, typical of such rooms where doctors eventually arrive (after what seems to be an interminably long time) to see their patients. The nurse closed the door, so now I had to prepare mentally for what I would say, and how I would say it.

After what seemed to be an eternity, the door abruptly opened and Dr. Wilkins entered. He wasn't smiling and after we shook hands, he folded his arms, looked at me with steely eyes, and said, "All right, tell me your story". I proceeded to speak. He asked no questions. I handed him the written reports and pointed to the scans I brought.

As he started reading, I broke in with a question. He politely but firmly let me know he'd rather I wait, so he could give his undivided attention to the reports. When he finished reading, quickly it seemed, he displayed the MRI scans. He said he would make his decision later. I left to return to Summerville. I had given it my best shot.

The four neurosurgeons we had encountered so far were all very professional. They were not unfriendly, but so caught up with their multiple responsibilities, so involved in the grim business that tumors created, that little opportunity existed to display a soft side, let alone empathy.

I recall taking Bobby once to a neurosurgeon for examination. I had been informed ahead of time that there would be a charge of one hundred dollars for the examination and the idea was for me to come prepared to pay. At some point during the examination, I gathered my courage and asked the doctor, "Why is it that neurosurgeons, as a class, do not display much in the way of sympathy or concern for either the patient or "God's Caregivers"? He really never answered, though he did give me a quizzical look. At any rate, when the exam was concluded, I went to the exit desk and prepared to write the check for one hundred dollars. The receptionist informed me, "The doctor says there will be no charge". Whether my simple question caused that result, I'm not sure. Or, it could have been a case where the doctor felt that he hadn't done that much and wasn't really in a position to help Bobby.

One of the few occasions in which I remember a neurosurgeon smiling was when we brought Bobby back to Children's Hospital in Philadelphia to have his stitches removed. Dr. Schute turned to me and said, "Well, I think it's time to remove Bobby's sutures". To which I replied, "Well, suture self". That evoked a smile after a startled reaction.

After Bobby died, I sent copies of the "In Memoriam" eulogy to over fifty persons who knew Bobby or knew of him. Dr. Perot wrote a lovely letter, in which he stated that the eulogy revealed to him a side of Bobby that he never had known. I thanked him and, in turn, pointed out to Dr. Perot, that his letter had revealed a side of him that we had not been aware of. Dr. Alfred Nelson, as well as several others, made contributions to The National Neuro-fibroma-tosis Foundation, Inc., in honor of Bobby.

Back in Summerville, we awaited word from Duke with a sense of urgency and uncertainty. Again, I finally took the bull by the horns and called Dr. Wilkins' secretaries, pleading for some kind of action. They said they'd see what they could work out.

Within a few days, we had a call. Bring Bobby to Duke. He would be admitted to Duke Hospital for unremitting pain and for several days of testing and evaluation. After which, Dr. Wilkins would make his decision—to operate or not to operate. As always, it was in God's hands.

Jane, Bobby and I took off for Duke, the first of five more weekly round trips for Jane and me of a good five hours driving time each way and five hundred fifty miles per round trip. Fortunately, my brother Armin stayed at our house when all this was developing, looking after Nicky, who was still ambulatory, but needed assistance in many areas of daily living.

After seeing Bobby admitted to the hospital, we stayed overnight, came by his room the next morning to see him, and then returned to Summerville to wait for the final decision.

On Friday, Dr. Wilkins said he would operate and believed that he had identified two tumors at the base of the spine as the ones causing his leg paralysis.

For five weeks, Bobby was in the hospital recovering. We felt that he would be in good hands, both remembering Duke from earlier years. When I returned home from Europe at the end of World War II, Jane was at her parent's home in Rocky Mount, North Carolina, only an hour's drive from Duke. We drove over there for Jane to have a physical checkup and her care and treatment were excellent.

What we were experiencing now was an entirely different attitude at Duke. Because of Jane's obligations at work and Nicky to look after, we traveled back and forth once a week. Usually staying overnight for several nights and seeing Bobby for two to three days.

While there, we fed Bobby, kept the hospital room as clean and straight as possible, and went looking for help when his call button went unanswered, which was often. A shortage of aides existed, and we sensed and observed a lack of concern for Bobby and an almost immediate response to black patients. We were encountering what appeared to be reverse discrimination and we were there often enough during the five-week stay to see that the situation was consistent. We hated to leave him, because when we did, it got worse.

One day, we began a conversation with a female employee. Chills traveled up and down my spine when she said that there was no way that she would leave a loved one of hers alone on that ward. The aides were running the place (we ran into this same situation later in a Low County nursing home). They were always short handed, overworked, and underpaid, and took it out on the patients, who were especially vulnerable when none of their family was around.

One Saturday afternoon, at about 3 P.M., we called Bobby to ask him if he had been given his bath yet. He said that he had not and that no one would respond to his repeated calls for help. We called back immediately and asked for the charge nurse. A woman came on the line, identified herself to Jane as the nurse in charge and demanded to know, in a hostile manner, what we wanted. Jane fought to keep from raising her voice. Finally, the charge nurse snapped, "who do you think takes care of him when he craps in his pants"?

Outrage over the conduct of the floor staff filled us, along with disbelief that such a thing could be taking place at Duke Hospital, an institution looked up to and trusted by so many.

Since it was the weekend, we had to wait until the following Monday. I phoned and insisted on being connected to the charge nurse for that ward. We talked long enough to learn that the person we had talked to Saturday had falsely identified herself as the "nurse in charge", when in reality she was only a nurse's aide who had been neglecting and harassing our son. Among other things, telling him that we had been complaining about the general conduct of the aides assigned to his room and, as typical, taking it out on him, instead of discussing it with us during our weekly visits.

I told the real charge nurse politely, but *very* firmly, that, in our opinion, the treatment that Bobby was being given was coming very close to violating his civil rights and was certainly devastating to any patient, but especially to one trying to recover from very severe major surgery. I told her that, if it were to continue, we would be in touch with our attorney.

She listened carefully, then asked me, "Mr. Weeber, do you consider Bobby's treatment to be reverse discrimination"? My answer was that unless someone could come up with a better description of what was going on, and why, it seemed to fit the situation perfectly. She promised to look into our complaints and take steps to improve the situation.

At this point, we were half way through the five weeks of his hospital stay and from then on, things did get better. I obtained the name of the hospital president and have often been asked why we didn't bring the matter to his attention.

I began to ask question (of anyone I though could be helpful) as to why Duke Medical Center, which at one time was hailed as the "Mayo Clinic of the South", no longer was operating in a manner to deserve that reputation. Part of the answer apparently lay in the fact that Duke Medical Center now had formidable competition from several area hospitals, regional and local, which had sprung up or modernized their operations over the past ten years. These hospitals, like Duke, were state of the art, had the latest hi-tech equipment, outstanding staff and, almost as important, employed large numbers of minimum-wage workers. Now, more than one hospital was offering quality medical research and health care that had in the past been a Duke hallmark exclusively for decades.

Also, crucial to staffing a hospital with large numbers of service-type workers, was the existence of an adequate labor pool. This no longer existed because of "the new kids on the block". Underpaid nurse's aides gained a new measure of independence, for they could now easily walk out of one institution and quickly find work at another. They now could and did assert themselves. Civil rights advances also gave job protection to the antisocial, racial types, thus, making it harder to terminate them.

Tired from the weekly round trips grind, worrying about Bobby's neglectful treatment, the financial expenses of the overnight stays, plus the desire to finish out Bobby's recovery there as well as possible, we opted not to address the maltreatment issue with the hospital management. We were also not anxious for what we expected to be a traumatic confrontation.

Further, what could the hospital, or anyone else for that matter, actually do about it? The damage had already been done and one of two things would probably happen: an apology or a denial. In either case, Bobby, we as his parents, and the hospital were all in the same boat. The conditions were such that the best result to be hoped for was a temporary cessation of the abuse to Bobby, but the pattern was deep seated and is unlikely to change for the better in the foreseeable future, certainly not because we had the courage to take a stand, which we had already done to the extent possible.

We are not faulting Dr. Wilkins. He and his team did their best. As he explained after discussing the poor treatment after the operation, it was not an area of his responsibility. The series of paralysis, operation and recovery had finally come to a halt. Bobby never walked again.

We brought Bobby home on October 28th. My son-in-law, John Bell, met me at the Duke Hospital in Durham and helped load Bobby in the car for the trip back home to Summerville. He stayed at home with us for one night and the next day he was out of the frying pan and into the proverbial fire.

Prior to leaving Duke, their social services department began working to place Bobby in an appropriate rehabilitation facility. Duke's rehab program had no opening to take Bobby at the date of his scheduled discharge. Also, we really weren't thrilled at having him continue under the custody of Duke after his five-week ordeal in the hospital.

Two other options opened. One involved a Health South rehab facility in Florence, South Carolina. We had already visited there and they probably would have done as well as any other. But we would be facing a two hundred twenty mile round trip just to see him once a week and that would have to be on a weekend. Not a good situation for us.

The second option was to try and get him a bed at MUSC's Rehab Unit (actually, one floor in a wing of the MUSC Hospital).

The boys had already been seen by the Director, Dr. James Warmouth and he was familiar with their medical history. Bobby would be nearer to us—a forty-mile round trip and in what was a well-regarded facility.

Again, we were told that openings were limited, but as discharge time from Duke drew closer, we pleaded with Dr. Warmouth to admit him, in the mistaken belief that that was the only solution and that we were doing the right thing for Bobby. Finally, almost at the last possible moment, he agreed to admit Bobby. We felt it was our son's best hope—and maybe our last hope—that he would walk again.

From day one, the rehab team seemed eager to hammer into us that Bobby had to "show progress" or he couldn't stay in the program. His physical therapists made no effort to conceal her opinion. "Bobby does not belong in this program", she advised us early and often!

We were hurt and upset, wondering why Dr. Warmouth agreed to admit him, while the team seemingly couldn't wait to discharge him. Who was in charge? The Director, who admitted him, or the physical therapist who kept telling us he didn't belong?

During his five-week stay, there was the usual offensive and un-called for conduct, by a young, white male aide. His pattern of resentment and hostility had him "taking it out" on someone who was vulnerable. This is one of the many different kinds of abuse, which doesn't always involve physically hitting or striking someone, but can be just as destructive to the victim. Jane reported his actions (and in some cases, lack of action) to the charge nurse and an immediate attitude adjustment followed. When this kind of abuse first rears its ugly head, nip it in the bud. You need to find out who the employee's superior is and don't hesitate to condemn such action as totally unacceptable. You need to imply—without at first saying so—that serious consequences will prevail if it continues. Yes, retaliation could occur, but in most cases, the institution can't afford to let bad conduct continue.

Bobby was at the lowest ebb of his life, mentally and physically, when he was admitted to MUSC Rehab on October 29, 1990, the day following his discharge from Duke Hospital, and was apprehensive about a repeat of the miserable conduct he endured at Duke Hospital in his new environment. He was homesick, discouraged that he couldn't walk and on top of that, we heard a physical therapist at Duke state in our presence and so Bobby could hear him, "My opinion is that he will never walk again". We were shocked, Bobby was devastated, and we felt that it was utterly inappropriate for anyone but a doctor to make such a statement and even then, certainly not "shooting from the hip". After four major surgeries, at age twenty-eight, he was unable to walk, even with all that he had endured and in a situation with no hope and no one really wanted him.

In retrospect, I'm sorry that we did not see that he was in an impossible situation, that the likelihood of his getting any real help was very questionable and that everyone concerned would have been better off if we were to ask for his discharge and taken him home. In one sense, the physical therapist was probably right…he did not belong *in the program*, or, in fact, *in any program*, anywhere else. In this stage of what was left of his life, he belonged home. We thought we were doing the right thing, but it was a big mistake. The wonder is that he lasted five weeks and is a tribute to the kind of character that he consistently displayed of being cooperative, trying to do his best under conditions that few of us would care to endure.

As Bobby was being discharged, the assistant director, probably deciding that Bobby would indeed never walk again and wanting him to have a high degree of mobility and a chance at an active life, wrote a prescription for Bobby to be custom fitted for a power wheelchair. She wanted him to be able to get out on his own. We appreciated her thoughtfulness.

Unfortunately, almost nine months passed after leaving MUSC Rehab on December 5th before the wheelchair was delivered. By that time, his body structure had changed and the custom molding, designed especially for his back, did not fit.

Adjustments to the misfit were ordered, but by the time they were implemented, they were ineffective. The worst impediment to Bobby's ability to use the wheelchair was that his hands were losing what strength they had left to operate the wheelchair "joystick". Paraplegia was rapidly approaching quadriplegia. I wound up trotting beside the wheelchair, operating the control myself. When I relinquished my grip, the braking system for the wheelchair would cause it to come to an abrupt halt. Several times, it almost overturned and we narrowly averted this danger. We finally had to give it up. We used it in his room to sit in and type, but he was never able to get the use out of it that the doctor intended. Ironically, in a few short months, it was to be the indirect cause of a tragic accident that took place in our house and in the bedroom where both boys spent their days.

On December 5, 1990, Bobby was terminated from the MUSC Rehab Unit and we brought him directly home. This began our involvement with home health care agencies and their home health care aides. As of Fall, 1998, we had received services through six different home health care agencies and in excess of two hundred home health care aides. Bobby was incontinent and this added another dimension to his case. We secured a hospital bed for Bobby and one aide was supposed to take care of both boys, since both needed assistance—Nicky far less than Bobby. We stored the power wheelchair in the garage, bringing it into their bedroom when it was Bobby's turn to type. We set up a card table, with the legs resting on wooden blocks to elevate it and positioned the wheelchair until it was comfortable for him to type. To make the transfer from bed to wheelchair, we brought in a Hoyer Lift.

This device consisted of a heavy canvas swing, secured by heavy chains to an overhead steel trapeze fitting. It was supported by large metal feet, on rollers, and a pneumatic hand-operated pump to raise or lower the canvas sling, containing the patient in a prone position, as necessary. When transferring *from* the bed, the patient lays flat and was rolled onto the canvas sling; when transferred to the wheelchair, the patient remained in the sling and when leaving the wheelchair, the sling is hooked up to hold him.

An obvious concern was the possibility of the patient being "dumped" out of the sling as it was being raised high enough to clear any obstacles. Bobby was deathly afraid of this happening. We assured him that we were being very careful and that two persons would always be handling the transfer.

On June 12, 1991, around noon, he had completed typing and asked to be transferred back to his hospital bed. A male nurse's aide had assisted in the transfer earlier from his bed to sit in the wheelchair and type. His safety belt was on him. The aide's scheduled hours were over and he had departed.

Jane and I started working the Hoyer Lift pump without noticing his body position, to make certain that he sat as erect as possible and positioned as far back in the chair seat as he could go—and to our horror, he fell out of the canvas sling to the floor, hitting his back on the steel "feet" that supported the lift. We put a pillow under his head, called 911, and tried to comfort him and quiet his crying. Within a few minutes, an Emergency Medical team arrived and some firemen from a nearby fire station. After checking him for broken bones, they carefully lifted him into bed. It was now about 1 P.M.

He seemed not to be in pain and was able to talk coherently. It was such a difficult journey from where we live to the MUSC Medical complex that we tried to avoid it whenever we can. Around 5 P.M., I was talking with a friend in the medical supply business and he insisted that we needed to get Bobby to the MUSC Trauma Unit. He called for us, and made arrangements that called for us to leave at once.

When we arrived, a resident neurosurgeon started checking him. Dr. Perot, the chief neurosurgeon at MUSC and the boys' personal neurosurgeon, arrived shortly thereafter to monitor the situation himself. Bobby was delirious now, eyes rolling, head drooping, and hallucinating.

When Dr. Perot asked if Bobby had a Living Will on file with the hospital, we were genuinely alarmed. He was placed in intensive care, where they were able to stabilize him. They did an excellent job.

The next morning, Bobby looked much better. Scans showed a severe bruise on the spinal cord, which already had so many problems, it didn't need anymore.

Finally, after nine days, he was discharged on June 21st and taken directly to Eagle Landing Health Care Centre in Hanahan, South Carolina, about eight miles from our home in Summerville. In retrospect, what Bobby had exhibited upon admission to the Trauma Unit was a "panic" or anxiety attack. Regardless, the consensus was that he would be better off in a nursing home, needing skilled nursing care and more services than we were able to provide.

Working through social services at MUSC, arrangements were made and a bed obtained for Bobby. Eagle Landing was a relatively new facility, beautifully furnished. His stay would be covered by Medicare (at that time, they had no Medicaid beds). He was to be there for sixty days, the first twenty of which were covered one hundred percent by Medicare, then a substantial co-insurance amount to be paid for by us for the other forty days.

One June 21, 1991, he was admitted. One June 23rd, we received a phone call around midnight, advising us that Bobby was coughing up and losing blood. They were taking him to the nearest hospital in accordance with their policy. We arrived about thirty minutes after being notified. Our youngest daughter and her husband were in town from Greenville, South Carolina and they met us there. When we arrived, Bobby was in the emergency room, being stabilized.

A tentative diagnosis by the emergency room doctor was waiting confirmation by a procedure known as endoscopy. This consists of dropping a tiny "camera", attached to a string, down the patient's throat, into the abdominal area. A picture is thus obtained to prove or disapprove the ulcer as the source of the bleeding.

Dr. John K. Corless, an experienced gastroenterologist did the procedure. The ulcer diagnosis was confirmed and was to be the first of four endoscopies done on Bobby over the next nine months. In light of all that he had been through, the existence of a bleeding ulcer should have come as no surprise.

While Bobby at first dreaded having the camera dropped down his throat, he endured and was able to tolerate it better as further such procedures were done, making new friends at Baker Hospital along the way. Dr. Corless discharged him on March 2, 1992, with instructions to take Tagamet from then on, as a precaution.

Baker Hospital did not have Bobby's medical records and were thus at a disadvantage in treating him. Eagle Landing's orders were to take emergency patients to the *nearest* hospital and that was Baker. The fact that this was all taking place in the middle of the night did not help at all. Late that afternoon, since Bobby was not doing well, we began the effort to get him transferred to MUSC.

The resident neurosurgeon did not know Bobby or his history and it took a good bit of persuasion to get MUSC to agree to the transfer. Had Dr. Perot been available, we're certain, it would have gone much faster and a lot easier. One June 26th, he was admitted to MUSC and was doing so poorly, we feared for his life. Finally, I told a hospital executive that is was imperative he go into intensive care. He seemed to be slipping away again. At last, a vacancy opened up in the IC unit and he was placed there on June 28th.

A light touch of humor occurred as well. Bobby, delirious, told us that he saw Margaret Thatcher and Gorbachev in the room. When I repeated this to a hospital staff worker, she replied, "Good, maybe now we'll have peace in our time".

After nine days, he was discharged and readmitted to Eagle Landing Health Care Centre. His belongings had been stored, by agreement, and he was assigned a solitary room. During his stay, no other occupant was placed in his room. Once a confused resident mistakenly entered the room, not knowing what he was doing, got in the bed and started to go to sleep! Bobby called to alert the on-duty staff to come and lead the visitor to his proper room.

We rented a TV for the room and Jane, Nicky and I came every day. We picked up lunch en route and helped them with their meal. We would then leave, but Nicky would stay to watch the soap operas with Bobby. As a result, Nicky was a daily witness to the ill treatment given Bobby, a fact the aides were both aware of and resented, which showed.

The nursing home was chronically understaffed, a situation made even worse on weekends, when management was conspicuous by their absence. The room stayed dirty. Repeated requests to clean it up were either greeted with contempt or ignored (with the excuse that no one was available to do it).

I went to the Administrator again and again. A show of concern would ensue, and a trip to Bobby's room to take notes and apparently verify whether I was telling the truth or not. Nothing was ever done, his abuse and neglect continued unabated. The "team" of aides cursed frequently and Bobby was on the phone to us often, reciting the latest indignities that had been heaped upon him.

Instructions were given, that, when transferring Bobby or lifting him, a lift device be used. These directions were ignored and they jerked him around manually. On one occasion, they put his phone under his bed, where he could not reach it and turned off the ringer.

One day, while Bobby was talking to his younger sister, Mary, calling from Atlanta, she overheard a nurse yelling at Bobby. Mary told Bobby to put the nurse on the line and Mary asked her, "Can't you please be decent to my brother"? The nurse responded to the effect that, if Mary were there, "I'll kick your ass". The conversation terminated at that point and Mary called back and spoke with the Administrator. To her credit, the nurse was fired within a few days.

Bobby had diarrhea most of the time he was there. We believe it was caused, at least in part, from the terrible living conditions in the nursing home, along with the medicine he was given to keep him quiet and asleep at night.

One male aide was outstanding, speaking up for Bobby, and telling the female aides to stop mistreating him and to stop transferring him without using the lift device. Everyone on his ward was calling for him, because he cared for all the patients. But the rest of the aides tried to make it appear that Bobby and Nicky were causing their resentment and they were "put on report" because Jane and I went to the management about it.

We pulled Bobby out ten days earlier than scheduled, because of the rotten treatment. Shortly thereafter, Charleston, South Carolina's TV-2 aired segments on two consecutive nightly newscasts, detailing ill treatment at Eagle Landing Health Care Centre.

Looking back, nothing positive was accomplished for Bobby's well being and his stay only confirmed what we had long suspected—that conditions similar to what Bobby was subjected to are likely to be found in most nursing homes. To an extent, that's true. But his experience had to be nursing home care at its very worst. An out-of-state, unresponsive and uncaring ownership set the tone for their operation. The aides went on strike suddenly, demanding a raise in pay. They were promised more money, but I don't know whether they ever got it.

We were required to make an advance deposit of two thousand, five hundred dollars, to cover amounts not paid for by Medicare. About sixty days after leaving, we received a return of the entire deposit. This was not due to any generosity on the part of Eagle Landing, but because we had excellent secondary coverage. People familiar with the physical appearance of the building and with the interior decorating and furnishings, found it hard to believe that conditions within could have been as bad as we found them.

We put up with it too long and should have contacted the South Carolina Nursing Home Advocate, as well as top management at the nursing home's corporate headquarters up North. We tried to be cooperative, hoping it would work out and the substandard conditions would be corrected. These were mistakes on our part and we have vowed never to let it happen again.

A good nursing home is no place for any patient to be confined, especially a younger person with a decent mind and the ability to express him or herself. A poorly run nursing home is absolute hell—for all patients!

For Bobby, the final earthly chapter was fast approaching, although he didn't know it and we didn't realize it—at the time. After all, wasn't there always one more operation, one more last chance at a decent life? Late in 1992, one of the better home health aides that we've had called our attention to a sizeable lump at the base of Bobby's spine. All of us checked it daily for several weeks—it seemed to be slowly increasing in size. We then called our doctor to come examine it himself.

He diagnosed a muscle mass and prescribed Valium. I had reservations, but we went along, looking at it frequently.

About the middle of February, I told our doctor that the muscle mass was getting alarmingly larger and Valium did not appear to be the answer. My words were: "Given the boys' history of tumors, the disease, and especially Bobby's multiple operations for tumor removal, it has to be a tumor".

We attempted to make an appointment with a neurosurgeon nearer to where we lived. He had Bobby's medical history, hand delivered to his office, by me, for about ten days. At the last minute, the day before the appointment was to take place, we were informed that he had decided not to see Bobby. The reason offered was that the hospital he was connected to "did not have the facilities" to handle this case.

On February 17th, we obtained an order from our family doctor to take Bobby to Trident Regional Medical Center in North Charleston, for a scan. We spent five hours in a hospital corridor, waiting for a CAT scan.

During this time, many different thoughts and feelings came and went—their presence unseen and unknown to Bobby, but very evident to me. My heart and mind were heavy with a multitude of thoughts, none of which were reassuring. I forced myself to make small talk with Bobby, avoiding discussion of topics that I felt would upset him if voiced.

FEAR was there. Fear that his scan results would confirm the existence of an enlarged tumor. Fear that it would be attached to or in very close juxtaposition to his spinal cord. Meaning, if that were the case, that no operation would be possible and his imminent death inevitable.

GUILT was there. Guilt that I wasn't forceful enough with his doctor. Insisting that a scan be done much earlier, when the lump was first discovered.

SADNESS overwhelmed me. The thought of losing Bobby became unbearable. I loved him very much and also knew that his passing would be incredibly hard on his identical twin brother, Nicky. And indeed, the intervening months and years have proven this concern to be true.

ANGER entered my consciousness. Bobby had suffered too much, with at least five major surgeries. The final injustice to him loomed large on the horizon.

RESOLUTION of Bobby's situation was small consolation. Yet we had to know, and above all, his doctors had to know exactly what his condition was, what they had to contend with and thus what his chances were. Their answers could mean that Jane and I probably would soon be presented with the hardest task that parents can be confronted with—telling your child that he was terminal and deciding when and how he had to be told.

The five hours spent dealing with these thoughts were among the most difficult hours I've ever had to endure.

Bobby was apparently unaware of the gravity of his situation. If he was concerned about it, he did not show any sign of it. He was more frustrated with the unusually long wait we both had to contend with. At his urging, and because I could see how uncomfortable he was lying on a hospital bed in a corridor with remodeling going on, I went several time to the department head to find out the reason for such a long delay and to request that his test be give as soon as humanly possible.

I eventually was told that his doctor's order called for an MRI (Magnetic Resonance Imaging). After some consultations back and forth, it was determined that a CAT scan would serve the purpose better. This, together with the remodeling, combined to cause the five-hour wait.

There is not guarantee that, given similar circumstances, this tragedy won't be repeated, should Nicky be stricken with an ordinarily benign tumor that suddenly decides to metastasize. We pray it won't happen.

The next day, our doctor gave us the news—the reading of the scan confirmed the location and existence of a sizeable tumor. My heart sank and I told Jane, feeling that in all probability, we would lose Bobby. Previous experience, plus the just announced finding, pointed heavily in that direction.

There was another—and last—shoe to drop. I called Dr. Perot on February 22nd with the news and we went immediately to MUSC so that Bobby could be seen both by Dr. Perot and Dr. Paul H. O'Brien, cancer surgeon and specialist. The two doctors looked down on Bobby as he waited expectantly. It seemed as though he was a Christian awaiting the verdict of Roman Emperors. Thumbs up? Thumbs down?

They came to a decision quickly. They simply could not operate because the tumor was attached to his spinal cord. It was in every sense of the word a death sentence—terminal. Bobby did not pick up on exactly what decision had been reached or how serious this was.

We returned home, trying not to show our heartbreak. We had to tell him, we owed him that, no matter home traumatic it would be for all of us.

At one point, Bobby said to me, "I'll be so glad when this tumor goes away, it hurts so bad when I'm sitting in the wheelchair, trying to type".

Upon arriving home from MUSC, we realized that we didn't know—hadn't been told and hadn't asked—how long he had to live. I called the next day and was told the prognosis was sixty days. That would have been April 22nd. He died of cardiac arrest on April 3, 1993.

In a mortal sense, the play was over…the final curtain had come down. We looked at him in the emergency room, lifting the sheet that covered him. Locked in the throes of rigor mortis, trying not to see the grotesque appearance that the giant tumor had created, literally crushing the life out of him, but to see him as God's child, free of earthly pain and torment, home again.

I bent and kissed his forehead, choking back the tears. "We'll meet again, Bobby", I said. I pulled the sheet back over him and left the room.

During the first week following his passing, Bobby appeared to me twice. On both occasions, the circumstances were the same. It was night, I was lying in bed, looking up at the ceiling, thinking about my son. Suddenly, his face was visible, surrounded by a shroud of white fabric. I said, "Bobby is it you"? "Yes", he replied. "Don't grieve for me, I'm fine". Then he was gone.

A few days later, the same event took place—the same words. Some will say it was the imagination of a distraught father. But I'm sure I did see him and he spoke to me.

WHAT WE LEARNED FROM THE RIDE ON
THE MEDICAL MERRY-GO-ROUND

Our "ride" has slowed down considerably, but events keep it turning. We recall the advice given us by our then family doctor in York, PA. He told us: "Sometimes you have to rattle your doctor's chains to get his attention".

When hesitant to speak up, if the occasion warranted it, we remembered his words and I guess we've done our share of "chain rattling".

We believe it accomplished the desired results, and while we may have raised some eyebrows, we don't recall ever losing any doctors because of it. We heartily recommend it!

CHAPTER FOUR

Education For The Learning Disabled

As soon as Bobby and Nicky were diagnosed as having neuro-fibroma-tosis, we quickly learned that a synonym for that was "learning disabled". As long as the boys were in a private, pre-school situation, they would be fairly well sheltered from abusive peers, classroom disruptions, and uncaring teachers and aides whom they would soon encounter in almost any public school system.

We placed them in a pre-school facility in Arlington, a suburb of Jacksonville, Florida, known as "The Little House in the Forest". They did reasonable well during their few years there, considering that no great demands were made on them—or, for that matter, on any of the children. You could honestly say that, in an educational context, their time in "The Little House" was like the "days of innocence" that we compare with today's brutality and mindlessness in the classrooms.

Not only was little known about neuro-fibroma-tosis in the early 1960's, special education programs for learning disabled students—and other, more serious classes of the physically and mentally disabled—were just being installed, or in many cases were non-existent.

After several years of pre-school, at the age where they had become eligible for public school, they were registered for enrollment in an elementary school nearest to where we were living.

In a year or so, a Special Education program for Duval County Schools was announced. We promptly applied to have them transferred to the nearest school where classes were to be conducted. After testing, they were placed in the Windy Hills Elementary School. They were just getting started when I received a job offer in York, Pennsylvania. I accepted the position, contingent on there already being in place a Special Education program in the York County, Pennsylvania School System.

We left Jacksonville, Florida and arrived in York, PA in May 1970. We were then told that such a program did not presently exist!

Thus began what was to be years of turmoil for the boys, as well as for ourselves. We finally were advised that a Special Ed program would be in place when school began in the fall. There was a Director in charge for York County, but we soon learned that he would be leaving. Internal dissension was already taking place.

In the works was the creation of "Intermediate" Units, designed to administer the Special Ed program statewide on a multi-county basis. Lincoln Intermediate Unit No. 12 was located in New Oxford, Pennsylvania, about halfway between York and Gettysburg. Their jurisdiction was three counties, including York County. There was a Director, Assistant Director, and a staff of psychologists and administrative specialists. They did not take over the administration of Special Ed programs until sometime later.

As a prerequisite to admission, Bobby and Nicky were tested and evaluated by the York County program psychologist. Bobby was accepted but Nicky was not. Their intelligence level was the issue. Because there had never been, to our knowledge, any appreciable difference between Bobby's intellect and Nicky's, we quizzed Nicky to see what the problem was. He told us that the psychologist was unfriendly, physically pushed and intimidated him. "I was afraid of him", Nicky told us.

I went to the York Suburban School District psychologist (the boys would be attending a school in that district) and found that she had the same opinion that Nicky did and that we did about the boys being of equal mental ability. Further, that they were identical twins and especially at their present age, should not be separated. She tested Nicky and found him acceptable, thus avoiding what would have been a desperate situation (no place for Nicky). The beginning was not encouraging—a harbinger of things to come!

Somewhere around 1975, they were passed on to a Junior High School in the York Suburban School District. At this level, no attempt was made to integrate the Special Ed students such as Bobby and Nicky into the so-called "normal" or regular classes.

The Special Ed students were in their own classrooms, with a male teacher and a female teacher's aide (at least that was the combination in their particular classroom). The boys began telling us about behavior on the teacher's part that could only charitably be described as bizarre. He was charging them to go to the bathroom; also taking things from them that they had brought from home and demanding money to give them back. In addition, he constantly yelled at them, criticized them and acted in a hostile manner, especially toward them. The teacher was frequently admonished about his conduct by the school's assistant principal.

I contacted the Director of Lincoln Intermediate Unit No. 12 to ask how such conditions could be allowed to continue. I was told that they were aware of the misconduct and gross behavior, but the teacher had "tenure" (meaning that he had been employed long enough to have attained certain "rights", including the right to a hearing and protection against being terminated without a hearing). The Director explained that they wanted to avoid a costly legal battle and were trying to negotiate an agreement with him that would, in effect give him a "clean" release and allow him to be passed on to another employer, without any of the misconduct being revealed. I was further informed that my complaints about his misconduct (made on behalf of our sons and all other students in that class) were upsetting him and would jeopardize their efforts to remove him from his position if I didn't cease and desist, so would I please stop commenting about him or to him, or confront him in any way!

While all of this was going on, the teacher wrote me a note, insisting that I come to a meeting with him. In view of what I had been told and because I sincerely felt that nothing could be gained by such a meeting, I did not respond. To meet with him would have been a mistake.

The school year ended and the boys were to report to a classroom in the Senior High School the following term. I later learned that the Lincoln Intermediate Unit had secured the teacher's resignation, given him a release letter, and that he was employed by a Federal Agency in Washington, DC. All things considered, it seemed like an appropriate disposition of the matter.

The Special Ed classroom at York Suburban High School was new when the boys reported in the fall. The York Suburban School District was rated as the "cream" of York area school districts, operating schools you would not only want your children to attend, but go out of your way to see that they did. The era of teenage rebellion was just beginning and lax administration compounded the problem. We were told that seniors cursed and derided the Superintendent and Principal in open assembly and were said to have smeared feces on some of the inside walls. And these were York County's "finest"!

The intent here was to "mainstream" as many Special Ed students into some "regular" classrooms as possible. Whether it was because the program had been poorly presented to the regular classroom teachers or whether, among the Special Ed students there were some with anti-social, discipline, or behavioral problems, dumped in with the merely learning disabled, I'm not sure. But "mainstreaming" never got off the ground, attributed to the disruptive conduct of a few, for whom there apparently was no other place to go.

A male student was brought into the boys' Special Ed classroom that was just such a type. He launched a daily litany of cursing, threatening to rape the teacher and her aide, as well as pulling out a sizeable switch-blade knife and telling Bobby and Nicky that he was going to kill them.

The teacher and aide put their own spin on it, saying, "It was only a little hat pin that couldn't even cut butter". That was their way of handling it!

The teacher had difficulty coping with what was going on. She and the aide presented a classic case of denial about a situation that would not have been easy for a physically strong, mature male teacher to deal with.

I went to the Superintendent (who had supposedly been a Special Ed teacher himself earlier in his career) and related what was taking place in the classroom and the demonstrated inability to do anything about it. I requested a hearing, saying to him, " You can't hate me for wanting to look after the welfare of my sons, can you"? He agreed that he couldn't and said he would take steps to set up a hearing on the issue.

Since no one with the establishment wanted to believe the boys or offer any support, I took the matter to a Trustee of the school board, who happened to be a member of our church, and selected Nicky to tell their story. We went to his factory, of which he was the owner, and Nicky related the details of what was happening, on a daily basis. I asked him, "Do you believe that Nicky is telling you the truth about this"?

He said that he did. He then asked me, "Do you feel that the Superintendent is unable to be objective about this business"? "So far, he has not indicated to me that he is", I replied.

Before the hearing, I found an attorney who was interested in specializing in "Education Law". I went over the facts with him and he agreed to represent us, pro bono, for the experience and to attend the hearing with us. Bobby stayed at home with Jane. Nicky had prepared a statement, citing events that took place and the dates they occurred, which he read at the hearing. The disruptive student did not attend. Incidentally, this boy came with a long history of infractions of discipline and brushes with the law.

The night of the hearing, Nicky and I walked in with the attorney, and I introduced him. From the look on the Superintendent's face, it was obvious that we had caught him by surprise. He seemed to be groping for some kind of response — I'm sure he was thinking "law suit". Finally, he advised us that tape recorders would not be permitted. I was happy to have an advocate in our corner, someone on *our* side.

The teacher and her aide were there and made a statement that, like the three monkeys, they saw no evil, heard no evil, and there was no evil, no big deal. Just a hatpin—couldn't even cut butter.

Our attorney made a strong statement, in an almost emotional voice, pointing out to the Superintendent that Bobby and Nicky, as well as all of the others in their class had a right to receive an education, free from intimidation and harassment on a daily basis.

I challenged the Superintendent to name one other classroom in all of York County where such behavior, taking place on a daily basis, was tolerated. He remained silent.

Then he accused me of wanting to place the offending student in a class for the socially and emotionally disturbed (this class was held at another school location). I replied that it was not my place to say where or in what kind of class he should be placed in…that was his job, along with the LIU staff. I did say that the one thing I was positive of was that he was not in his right place.

The meeting adjourned. At some point, the boy left school and I don't know what became of him. He had little or no parental support, no one who cared enough about him to tell him right from wrong.

Another incident took place before the hearing. An Assistant to the Superintendent had been hired and the understanding was that he would be named Superintendent several years down the road, when the incumbent took retirement. I asked him to meet with me; I met him at a restaurant where we had a clandestine discussion, during which conditions in the boys' classroom in particular, and the school in general, were brought out by me. I told him that the Principal was of no help, continually stating, in response to the boys' reports of misconduct, "I'll look into it", then taking notes and never doing anything about it.

He indicated that he couldn't do much about it, but promised to visit our sons' classroom and observe, which made the teacher and her aide suspicious. The teacher asked the boys if they had anything to do with his visits, which of course they denied. This went on for several months—then suddenly he was gone!

Knowing what the boys went through, and being a witness to most of it, I admire what they were able to accomplish—against the odds of the bureaucratic educational system and the jeers and sneers of their peers. The girls were the worst and the boys' rides on the school bus got so unpleasant that I often wound up taking them to school in the morning and getting them home in the afternoon.

Some good teachers along the way cared and did their best. And the boys made a few friends. But all of the activities that could have made school at least bearable, such as driver's ed, sports, proms, music, art, etc., they were ruled unable to participate. In some instances, they probably could not handle the activity, but it was always assumed they wouldn't fit in and in many cases, the teachers were afraid to have any Special Ed students in their classrooms.

Bobby and Nicky finally graduated in 1982. They received a diploma, stating that they had met the requirements of the Special Education program. We were told that they could remain in school one more year, to age twenty-one. After a short discussion with them, we agreed with them that they had had enough.

(Because of what they had seen and encountered since entering the public school system, it became impossible to get the boys to accept the fact that many young people graduate from high school, then go on to college, or other institutions of advanced learning, voluntarily, paying for all or at least a part of the cost themselves, for the privilege of obtaining a higher and better education). That the climate for learning was much better, having eliminated most of the rock heads and smart alecks who were too dumb to see the value of a decent schooling.

Several years after their graduation, I did persuade them to take a sixteen-week typing course at York Vo-Tech School. I took them in the early evening, twice a week. After several weeks, I noticed that the papers they were bringing home looked pretty darn good. I asked them if they were looking at what they were to type or looking at the typewriter keyboard. Their answers were not clear, so I called the teacher and asked him. He said he didn't know, but would watch them and let me know. A few days later, he called to tell me that they were looking at the keys, which explained why the papers looked so good. They finished the course, but a final typing test showed that their score of twenty-five words per minute, corrected, was three words per minute *less* than they typed before entering the class! So much for higher education!

When the boys reached eighteen, we decided to take them for counseling, mainly to get a third party point of view into their thinking. After all, up to this point in their lives, they had heard primarily from us on personal matters and we truly hoped that good counseling could bring new ideas and a new perspective on things to Bobby and Nicky. The "birds and bees" were part of it, but we also hoped that the counselors would give them some input on dealing with antagonists, immature persons in general, their own sexuality (or lack of it) and some things to look out for in dealing with others.

We had already found an excellent agency and an honest, capable counselor and started taking the boys to him on an every two-week schedule. After a while, it worked out better for him to come to our house and he and the boys would have lunch. Bobby and Nicky were encouraged to state their true feelings, vent anger, even cuss if they felt like it. The young counselor wore a heavy beard. I figured that he did so to identify with his clients, many of whom were borderline psychotics and came from a class of persons best described as "the great unwashed".

After a while, he suggested that we try a guidance service, to get the benefit of their expertise. Jane's insurance would cover part of it and it seemed like it might be a step forward in the process of giving the boys a healthier understanding of both themselves and others.

For a month or so, things seemed to be going well at the Guidance Clinic. Then, both boys began to tell us about one-hour sessions where the two counselors (one for each boy) spent three quarters of the hour either on the phone with other clients, visiting with each other, going for coffee, or on the phone talking to each other, while the boys were sitting in the offices wondering what was going on. At this point, we then called for a conference to find out their explanation.

Knowing that it would probably be the two "guidance" counselors against the boys' version, we invited the capable counselor who had worked with the twins for several months to sit in on the conference and even the odds for a fair deal.

My wife, our sons, their original counselor, and myself were present, as were the two guidance clinic counselors as the conference began.

After a few opening remarks, Nicky, the least likely spokesperson, delivered a concise, devastating statement that outlined the displeasure and anger that he and his brother felt with what had been going on. He said "Moe and Ike spend most of their time on the phone with other clients, each other, or going back and forth from one to the other, drinking coffee and goofing off. We're lucky to get fifteen minutes of counseling out of an hour. On top of that, we're not allowed to voice our opinions. There is an apparent obsession with sex, showing us pictures of naked women and telling us to just do it. That's not why we're here". Slamming his fist down on the conference table, he said, voice rising, "This shit has to stop or we're not coming back"! When his fist hit the table, everyone flinched and the guidance counselors jerked back in their chairs. The head honcho said to Nicky, "Are you saying you're not coming back"? Nicky replied, "If we're going to be ignored, not be permitted to express our feelings and you guys keep goofing off, why should we come back"?

The conference adjourned and we felt like cheering for Nicky. It was absolutely his finest hour! Later, one of the boys overheard the guidance guys arguing with each other. The head guy said, to his assistant, "You almost cost us the account—you better watch out"!

Later on, the head counselor told Bobby, "Well, your brother did a good job"! To which Bobby responded, "He did a damned good job"!

After a few weeks though, we withdrew both boys from the sessions. So much for the birds and the bees!

WHAT WE LEARNED ABOUT EDUCATION FOR THE LEARNING DISABLED

There are many labels that are often placed on children who are not "up to par" in their school- work. "Brain damaged" and "learning disabled" are the most common. It is important that YOU make sure that the person doing the labeling knows what they're doing.

If an educator or school psychologist makes the identification, it is wise to go to your pediatrician or family counselor for confirmation. If it's your doctor, see the school administrator NOT the school nurse or teacher.

When your heart knows that things are not right for your student, don't be afraid to challenge authority. YOU must act as the ADVOCATE for your child.

*Remember, thousands of men and women have gone through life successfully at every level and never knew that **they** had a learning disability. Just think what that means!*

CHAPTER FIVE

Religious Faith—
A Powerful Force In Our Lives

Looking back on fifty-six years of marriage—even as I write this—especially the fifty-two years following the birth of our first daughter, Wanda, we cannot claim to be an overly religious family.

Although Jane and I were married in a Baptist Church in Jacksonville, Florida, by a Baptist preacher, we soon decided that we needed a church home in which both of us would be comfortable. Her father was a Baptist preacher in North Carolina. He attended Wake Forest College, when it was in the town of Wake Forest, NC. I was raised in Christian Science, my mother's influence, while my father was more an agnostic than he was an atheist. For a while, he attended Christian Science services and seemed to find the help he was looking for, but eventually stopped going and reverted to his former state of doubt.

I could see that Jane would have a difficult time accepting Christian Science, given her background, while I felt equally uncomfortable with the Baptist theology. We had no trouble agreeing on the Presbyterian faith. We joined the Arlington Presbyterian Church in Arlington, Florida (a suburb of Jacksonville, Florida).

We have continued in the Presbyterian Church ever since. All of our children have attended Sunday school and all of the four have gone on to become Presbyterian Church members.

The boys were eight when we arrived in York, Pennsylvania, in 1970. Mary was eleven. For two years, we attended Eastminster Presbyterian Church and in 1972, we joined by transfer of our letter from Florida.

Unfortunately, the same treatment of harassment and hostility they got in public school was also evident in the Sunday school classroom. A church member, volunteering to help out as an aide in the boys' classroom, saw what was going on and would lovingly sit with the boys to shield them from the taunts and hateful remarks. Thus began a friendship that has endured to this day, over ten years after we left York!

The minister was probably unaware that un-Christian conduct was taking place in the boys' Sunday school classroom. "Teachers" were often not present and even when they were, most had little or no training in how to cope with unruly and restless youngsters, many of whom didn't really want to be there to begin with.

In general, the church was very supportive. Three elders especially stand out. They either taught Sunday school classes or were church leaders. Steve Beach, Jim Stine, and Bill Kirk were the three, whose love and concern for the boys has also extended and continued through the years.

Bill Kirk has been outstanding, remembering both boys on their birthday and at Christmas, with phone calls at intervals throughout the year. When their confirmation year came up, Bill helped arrange for them to tape their affirmation of faith, which they wrote themselves and played back before a full church audience. It was very effective and well received.

Bobby and Nicky volunteered to stock the pews in between weekly services with various printed items.

Upon moving to Summerville, South Carolina, in 1988, Jane, the boys, and I joined the Summerville Presbyterian Church. Because of their worsening physical condition, they were unable to attend services.

The membership and all of the ministers have taken an interest in the boys and have given their support in many ways. A succession of a retiring minister, an already retired minister, a resigned minister, and a parish associate minister, as well as a minister who left to lead his own church, and a newly appointed minister, brought six ministers into our lives during a seven year period! One minister, having left to lead his own church, came to our house at infrequent intervals to bring lunch and enjoy a *Star Trek* video episode with the boys. He continued, after receiving special permission, even after being appointed minister of his own church, many miles from here, but finally was unable to keep coming.

Jane Weeber passed away September 10, 1999. She truly devoted a major portion of her life to our twin sons.

WHAT WE LEARNED ABOUT FAITH

We have often been asked, "How did your faith help you on a daily basis? Really help you to get through?"

After giving it thought, I'd have to say that our answer has everything to do with the commitment we've made to our sons, i.e., to keep them at home, look after their well being, keep them out of a nursing home—and the challenges we faced on an almost daily basis in doing so.

When the going gets rocky, and we find our ability to cope with the problems and disruptions diminishing with our advancing years, a sense of responsibility kicks in and our duty comes into sharper focus.

In effect, the act of "keeping the faith" with our sons is the mechanism that calls forth faith itself to see us through. We know, through a constant supply of faith—where, when and as needed—that there is only one source for it, and that it is a gift from Him.

There have been—and still are—countless times when both of us believe that we simply can't face another day, even begin to question our commitment and resolve. We're on our knees mentally, if not physically, asking that the strength we need be renewed, and He has never failed us.

CHAPTER SIX

Dealing With Home Health Care Agencies
And Home Health Care Aides

Since bringing Bobby home from MUSC Rehab in early 1991, we have been involved with six home health care agencies and over two hundred home health care aides—and counting! It is therefore, understandable that the three of us (especially Nicky) have negative feelings about these figures. More so with respect to the aides than to the agencies they work for.

In every case where we were driven to leave an agency, it was because they could not provide home health care aides who were dependable, had a decent attitude, conducted themselves in a professional manner, or, too often, any aides at all.

For us, selecting an agency was somewhat restricted, depending on which entity would be paying for the service. Otherwise, there wasn't a lot to choose from, since they all had the same problems to contend with.

Every agency normally had an Administrator, almost always a female, and almost always a Registered Nurse. While a Registered Nurse might be excellent as a working RN, attending to her patients, it doesn't necessarily follow that she will be a good Administrator, the same way that an outstanding salesperson seldom makes a good sales manager.

We averaged about one and a half home health care agencies a year. They all had impressive "Patient's Bill of Rights" manifestos, setting forth their duties and responsibilities to their clients. It sounds good and reads great, but in most cases it amounts to rhetoric—and little more.

We had been with our fifth agency for a little over a year and a half. It was one of four agencies on an "approved" list (agencies approved by the Department of Disabilities and Special Needs, who provide the boys' services) and we had already been with two of the other three.

They started out well and while some of the aides were so unpleasant that we has to request that they not come back, some were excellent aides as well. However, from the first of 1996 to October, the operation began going downhill. Over their last four months, about twenty percent of the scheduled hours that we were entitled to were not fulfilled. For example, on a Friday night (too late in the week to do much about it) a newly scheduled aide who was supposed to work for us on that weekend, called and said that due to a personal emergency concerning her aunt in the mid-state section of South Carolina, she would not be able to come. The following was the result, for the three of us:

	SATURDAY		*SUNDAY*	
Schedule:	7:30 AM—1:30 PM	NO ONE	8:00 AM—Noon	NO ONE
	4:30 PM—6:30 PM	NO ONE	4:30 PM—6:30 PM	NO ONE

On the following Monday morning, our usually dependable morning aide phoned at 7:00 AM to say that her son needed emergency surgery and because she had to be with him, she could not come. We certainly understood. At that hour however, calling the agency would be futile. Nothing left but to pull ourselves together and do what Nicky needed done for him. That meant a total of nineteen hours that Jane and I bore the physical burden of doing for Nicky.

While this was the longest we had to go without help, in other ways it was more or less what we had come to expect. Last minute "bad news" phone calls, no replacements or backups in sight and not much concern for the predicament it left us in. Calling the agency had become almost useless, as they consistently were unable to send anyone when the scheduled person bombed out.

About all the agency could seem to come up with were two or three aides whose conduct was so reprehensible that, as badly as we needed help, we simply felt that we would be worse off if we allowed them to come back. We were then accused of being "picky", so it was our fault we wouldn't take the unacceptable aides as replacements. They were in fact what I call the dregs, which other clients also didn't want. Why else were they always the only ones available? But shifting the blame to us was convenient.

The "blessings" of downsizing have already filtered down to the home health care agencies. One of our past agencies is a case in point. Where before it had three offices, reasonably staffed, serving three major metropolitan markets, the operation was centralized into one office, with "token" staffing in the other two. A lot of jobs were eliminated and probably impressive sums of money were saved, but clients such as us, and aides have been hurt. We understand that now they are having second thoughts and a partial return to the former staffing is taking place. We didn't see any improvements in their ability to provide scheduled help or concern for ourselves others who find themselves in the same boat.

Only a limited pool of South Carolina State certified home health care aides is available. All agencies are contesting for new hires and all offer pretty much the same deal. In addition, hospitals, nursing homes, clinics, residential care homes assisted-living facilities and state agencies are competing for licensed persons, willing and able to work the hours given them.

What it boils down to is this: you take the neglect, the lack of concern, inability to staff your needs, failure to keep you informed, and failure to care very much about your loved one and the "God's Caregivers" involved, as long as you can stand it. Then, in desperation, you try yet another agency.

Several years ago, when we were calling every number we could get hold of, trying to obtain some kind of services for both boys, from whatever state agency might exist to provide this, we called an 800 number, the South Carolina Handicapped "Hotline". A very nice lady informed us that she had a handicapped daughter and, in two years, had been through over one hundred fifty home health care aides. I thought at the time that she surely must be exaggerating, but after what we have been through and are still going through, and will never be entirely free from the situation, I'm convinced now that she was telling the truth!

In fairness, not every problem with home health care can be blamed on the agencies. They are dealing with a difficult segment of society, either un-or under-educated for the most part, doing a dirty job for not a lot of money, and carrying a very heavy load of personal baggage.

Aides have been known to sign time sheets showing hours worked that they didn't. As a class, they are not dependable, although exceptions do exist. Also, some caregivers and/or patients are both demanding and unreasonable. Plus, competition is fierce for aides who can show state certification and a decent work record and most have no hesitation switching from one agency to another for one dollar an hour more.

HOME HEALTH CARE AIDES
(Also known as Personal Care Aides and Nurse's Aides)

Trying to evaluate the over two hundred aides we've had on an individual basis is difficult, if not impossible. They came (and went) in such numbers and so rapidly that we can't even recall a lot of their names. From the beginning, we should have kept a roster, but never dreamed we'd have such numbers to keep up with.

Conclusions about aides in general are a little easier to come to. Rating an aide on a scale of one to ten, we would come up with an average grade of six. The ones who were so obnoxious and lacking even elementary care and respect for the patient that we had to tell the agency not to send them ever again, would rate a one or two—and even, in more than a few cases, a zero.

The better aides, maybe a half dozen or so, would not rate a ten, as even they had some drawbacks. So, what would some of the factors be that it would be reasonable to expect of a certified nurse's aide (or personal care aide)? A few, not necessarily in the following order: Neat in appearance, pleasant manner (no sorrowful expressions), basic intelligence, a willingness to work, and physically able to do the work required. Able to follow directions and remembering to do the basic things that trial and error on our part have proven to be the best for all concerned—the patient, the caregiver and the aide. Not attempting to control, manipulate, or dominate the patient. No abuse of any kind, physical or mental. Respecting the patient and the caregiver. A caring attitude. Being reasonable in using the client's telephone or otherwise "taking over" the facilities in the client's residence. Being as kind and responsive to the patient when "God's Caregivers" are not on the scene as they are supposed to be when "God's Caregivers" are present. Refraining from discussing their religious faith or beliefs, or attempting to force them on the patient, regardless of whether well intentioned or not, especially when asked not to. Last, but not least: COMMON SENSE!

We are not naïve enough to believe that we will ever have an aide who will meet all of the above specifications. We know that we have had only a few who came close. And yet, in reality, nothing listed, should not be expected. No racial issues determine how good or what kind of an aide a person is. It is basically a woman's field…two male aides out of one hundred (if that many). Perhaps eight African-American and twenty white.

We have been accused of being racist, which is utterly without foundation. I will admit, however, that a few have been so rank and immature in their conduct, that they sorely tempt me with a racist's viewpoint. But I restrain myself and realize that that would not be fair to the overwhelming majority who don't provoke such feelings. The fact is that the aides who have performed the best—met more expectations—are mature, Afro-American women. We are proud that they really do care about Nicky, treat him with the respect that he's entitled to and also that they consider us as their friends. When they are on duty here, they are treated as part of our family. They have overcome most of their problems, to the best of their ability. We are grateful for them being here to help us and have never failed to let them know, by words and deeds.

Three aides have been with us at some point during the past five years. They are among those whom we hold in the highest regard. Three others were certainly not the kind we want back.

Now, the following three aides would be the first to tell you that they are far from perfect. Each have some qualities that we'd like to see changed or improved, but they all have several things in common, unlike the majority of aides. These qualities are—IN ORDER:

Responsibility/Dependability

We know that we can count on them to be here, on duty, if we are just a few hours away or in another city on twenty-four hour respite time. We trust them with the safety and well being of our son, whom we care about—and so do they.

Experience/Intelligence

Each has had years of home health care experience. They can and do work for more than one agency and they are in demand. They are mature, have and use common sense. We are confident that, in an emergency, they can and will react appropriately and promptly.

Caring

This is the one quality that is, in many ways, the most important. The one that, without which, other positive character traits by themselves alone are insufficient. They may not always agree with the patient and he may not see eye to eye with them. All either have children and grandchildren or are surrounded by family. They do care. And since you can't care deeply about someone without also loving him or her, we feel that they love Nicky too. They overlook his shortcomings and do their best to make their time with him as pleasant as can be.

As caregivers, working against the daily impact of our years on our abilities to care for our son, we feel that these aides, above all others, see what we are trying to do, i.e., keep Nicky at home with us (and out of a nursing home) and therefore, care about Jane and I as well.

CLARA FAILEY

Clara is from Johns Island, South Carolina and if you know anything about the Low Country, you are aware that life is rugged in that area. One has to be tough to make it and Clara is. On top of that, Clara served in the Army and still shows the effects of Army discipline. Yet, with it all, she has an underlying sensitivity and compassion. Once, when I questioned her about something concerning Nicky's care that wasn't going the way it should have, she did not take it too well, feeling that I didn't trust her. And if that were the case, she wouldn't be coming back. We got that cleared up.

When Bobby passed away, she was taking care of him. His death made an awful impact on Clara and I can honestly say that outside of Jane, Nicky, our daughters and myself, she took it harder and it lasted longer than anyone else. It was months before she finally felt able to come to our house to visit Nicky and chat with him. How do *you* define caring and love? We think she did that very well.

LATHESHA HOLT

Lathesha Holt came to us and showed the quality of love and caring, both for Nicky and for us, that was especially noteworthy in view of her situation and personal problems. To begin with, she is an LPN and started coming to us because the agency couldn't give her enough LPN rated clients. She was not happy about that. She is a single mother and was involved in a custody battle with her ex-husband. In addition, she is on her way to becoming a registered nurse. So here is a person with a huge load of personal baggage, but who never once took it out on Nicky.

She would forget some things (most of them minor) and often ran late, but her kindness and caring manner helped to cancel out the negative aspects. In addition, in many instances, she went to great lengths just to be here, knowing that if she didn't, we would have no one. Also, part of the equation: she got just two hours of pay (at the Certified Nursing Aide rate) for each visit.

She left us and also resigned from the agency. Tears flowed freely on her part and Jane's. She is sorely missed, but we are happy for her that she can go on, earn more money, and do the superb job she's proven she can do. She still keeps in touch and visits when she can.

MARY MYERS-DOLES

Mary was born in South Carolina. She has lived and worked in New York City. She is another single mother, with two grown daughters, a teenage son and another, younger daughter. In addition to her work as a home health aide, she takes her responsibilities as a mother and grand-mother seriously. Life in general and her, children have given her much to concern about.

She has done practically all of our respite time…those 24-hour peri-ods where we get away and she is on duty every hour until we return. It took a long time before Nicky would trust her to physically handle his necessary transfers (bed to commode, commode to power lift chair, etc.) *by herself.* She is strong and does the transfers with complete abil-ity and confidence that he will not be dropped to the floor.

Mary has gone out of her way to come back again, after her sched-uled hours here have been completed, as a back-up on her own initia-tive when the scheduled aides fail to show. And this has happened many times. She is a true friend, with Nicky's well being at heart.

Other aides have done outstanding work here. Many were so good that they deserved and often received promotions, meaning better pay and working conditions. We could almost tell when we were about to lose an aide and we usually were right.

Jane and I have *never* given any aide a direct order in a hostile or angry manner, or in any way at all, for that matter. Nor has Nicky ever done so. We all say "please" or "would you mind"? To get across those things that we must voice.

In the last few years, we have gotten so that we can almost always tell, by meeting and having a brief conversation with a new aide, whether they are going to work out or not. We've gone to ridiculous lengths in many cases to give it time "to work out". I am now going to profile a few case histories of aides whose entire manner made their remaining on the job here impossible. But, while unacceptable to us, in most cases agencies merely assign them to a different client.

#1

#1 was very high strung. As usual, she was sent to us at a time when the agency apparently had no one else. The first sign of trouble came when she started right in using our phone almost constantly. Her voice was loud and strident and her conversations were full of anger and hostility. When Jane finally had to ask her to cut down on the calls, she became very angry.

One night I offered to see here to her car, parked in the back of our house, on the other side of our fence. It was dark and we were concerned that something might happen to her. Before we could leave the house, she grabbed a switchblade knife out of her handbag, opened it, and then waved it around shouting, "This is my escort"! Later, she went to Nicky's room, pulled out the knife again and said, "You should have seen your father and mother turn white when I pulled this out".

Needless to say, we contacted the agency, relating the events and making it clear that we wanted her replaced *AT ONCE!* Amazingly, the agency did not seem to be overly concerned. A history of such behavior existed, only the agency looked the other way and merely passed her on to another client. I wouldn't be surprised if she was not working. Would you want a person with such a temperament caring for you, your loved ones or anyone you know?

#2

#2 came to us with a hearty recommendation, "She is where it's at...you'll love her". Unfortunately, she soon displayed indications of religious fervor, which we had found difficult to deal with before. One day, the aide informed the twins she was going to take them away from us and we would never see them again. She outlined how they would be taken to a place where we would never find them. Also, she intended somehow to gain control of their Social Security checks (I am and have been for many years, their Representative Payee).

She kept repeating the scenario to the boys, which indicated that the whole idea was rapidly becoming an obsession. On the face of it, the whole thing was bizarre and bordered on the ludicrous. Such events occur every day. Although she could well have just been blowing smoke, it is also true that where there's smoke, there's fire. So, we asked for an immediate replacement, attributing the reason to a "personality conflict" (to avoid possible retaliation).

#3

#3 was immature and had unrealistic expectations that seemed as though they had to have come out of a civil rights handbook.

She started off with the following routine, which we mistakenly put up with for three weeks. We didn't believe what we were seeing and foolishly thought it would soon stop, until finally we had to take a stand.

She would come in late to work each morning, looking and acting exhausted. After hurriedly going through the care sheet, she would come into our living room, plop down on a plush, swivel chair, turn on the TV—and fall asleep! Jane and I would look at each other, shake our heads, keep our voices down, tip-toe around, and do what had to be done for the boys.

Finally, I told her that it was inappropriate to take over the house and fall asleep and/or watch TV. That this was not what she was hired for.

(This seemed to come as an unwelcome revelation). I saw her to the door as she walked off the job, crying loudly as she departed.

Within several hours, the Agency Administrator was on the phone, asking me if I considered myself a racist and why didn't we report this kind of behavior sooner?

To answer the racist implication, I gave her the names of four aides, all African-Americans, as references we had no hesitation in naming as proof that there was absolutely no racial animosity by any of us, the boys included. Several had continued their contacts with us, years after they were no longer being assigned here.

As to why we didn't report her taking over the house and falling asleep watching TV, we said that we put up with it as long as we could, so we couldn't be accused of not "giving it time to work out". We heard no more about it and awaited the arrival of aide number fifty-something, wondering what next?

The last three I've profiled were about as unsuitable as they come, though many others came close. After seven years of encounters, we can tell you that you can take the following to the bank:

The only thing certain about dealing with home health care aides and their agencies is the guaranteed uncertainty of it. Just when you think you finally have the right people on the right schedule, something will come along to convince you otherwise.

It may be a new ruling by Medicare, Medicaid, or your private insurer; it might be a new policy by DHEC or perhaps your agency has made a change in operating procedures. But, you can count on it being *something* you have not anticipated, thought of, or experienced before.

Just when you're positive you've heard every reason or excuse possible, you will hear a new and different one—until the next time.

Our advice is: if an aide is obviously behaving in an inappropriate manner, no matter what the agency tells you, don't wait—insist that they be replaced at once. You are better off to have no one than someone who will abuse your loved one or take advantage of you, the caregiver.

After a while, you'll develop a "feeling" that will enable you to fairly accurately tell, the moment they step into the house and open their mouth, whether it's going to work out "right" or not.

Above all, never let an aide "take it out on a patient" (or you, for that matter). At the first sign of this, contact your Administrator and request—don't ask—that the person be replaced.

By this time, you may have concluded that unsatisfactory staffing arrangements (or in too many cases, no arrangements at all) are not always the fault of the agencies. They run recruiting ads, interview prospective aides, and make the best effort they can to sign up those whom they feel are worth it. References are checked, but not much more. Criminal background checks are normally not made. You really have no way of knowing whether you have a convicted felon working in your home or not. For example, out of the two hundred plus we've had working in and out of here, we're truly not sure, but out of that many, with no criminal background checks having been made, it wouldn't be surprising if one or two had some prior conviction on their records. The schools that offer courses for nurse's aides certification include ethics and professionalism instruction, but the results seem to indicate that, in most cases, it doesn't take. That's probably because unless you are raised to know right from wrong and the need for human beings to express compassion and show a caring heart, it's too late for a short course in a school to do the job.

Aides, after being assigned to a client, often either call the agency at the last minute to say that they can't make it, or in many cases don't call anybody. Also, if they do call in, the agency is supposed to let the client know right away, but often the person taking the call at the agency, simply doesn't follow through. If the agency has directed the aide to call them and not the client, the client and patient are left with no word. All of these possibilities have been too real for us in a number of situations.

We have gaps in our coverage, with the agency unable to find suitable persons to fill the need. According to several agencies, our location, twenty miles from Charleston, South Carolina, is such that, unless an aide happens to live in Summerville or close by, it is farther than they want to go. As a rule, they do not get mileage allowances. Another problem is that aides don't want to work on weekends, Also, if an aide has worked forty hours for one agency, they won't be allowed to work any more hours for that agency. As a result, many work for two or more agencies.

The last several years were especially hard on Jane and me. With so many hours unfilled, the burden has fallen heavily on us. People ask, "How's Nicky"? To which I reply, "He's fine, but his caregiver parents are hurting". To top that off, you eventually get that abandoned feeling, that nobody understands what it is really like and furthermore, that nobody cares! That's when we have to reach back and draw on our physical and mental resolve to stay the course, asking God to watch over and help all of us, as He always does. To believe that things will ease up, sooner than later, and generally they do. On Monday, November 11, 1996, *USA TODAY* started a series of reports on home health care abuses, Medicare/Medicaid fraud, and the following story: "Chronic Illness Takes Surprising Toll on Caregivers". The series ran through Wednesday, November 13th. Readers, already alarmed by congressional wrangling over Medicare, Medicaid, and Social Security, were not reassured by these disclosures. We were not surprised, having been the victims of many of the problems uncovered by the *USA TODAY* survey.

It only seem as though it has to get worse before it gets better. Medicare incompetence and lack of enforcement are responsible for many of the abuses.

WHAT WE LEARNED ABOUT HOME HEALTH CARE AGENCIES AND HOME HEALTH CARE AIDES

After dealing with six home health care agencies and over two hundred home health care aides (also known as nurse's aides) and counting—over a period of eight years, we feel reasonably qualified to share a few observations.

As far as agencies go, all face most of the same problems. All are competing for the same supply of aides, not only with each other, but also with large institutions like hospitals, nursing homes, etc. Treatment largely depends on the administrator and how they delegate responsibility and follow through. With all respect to registered nurses, we did not find that they generally make good administrators (in the same way that a star salesman doesn't very often make a good sales manager).

As far as aides go, they range from loving and caring to unpleasant and abusive. Not necessarily physically hurting anyone, but guilty of one or more traits of abusive conduct, some of which are more damaging than striking or slapping a patient.

You need to listen to your loved one and, within reason, encourage him or her to be assertive and that certain behavior and actions are unacceptable. If that fails, as unpleasant as it may seem to you, you need to call the agency head—NOT the person who does the scheduling—and insist that the aide be replaced at once, or as soon as possible. You and your patient are entitled to that, to the same degree that aides deserve decent treatment, because respect and dignity are due both parties.

CHAPTER SEVEN

Thoughts on Caregiving

Shortly after we arrived on the "Low Country", we joined the Summerville Presbyterian Church and not long after that word got around that we had identical twin invalids to take care of. That was in 1988. I was seventy and Jane was sixty-six. Neither of us is large physically and neither has ever been strong from a physical standpoint. At that time, we had just gotten home health care of fourteen hours per week, two hours a day Monday through Friday and four hours on Saturday; nothing on Sunday. That meant we were on duty twenty-two hours a day, Monday through Friday, twenty hours on Saturday and twenty-four hours on Sunday.

Our church membership is probably an average age of sixty, with many far older. They wanted to help, but looking at it from all angles, it didn't seem practical to accept the kind offer to help that many made. First of all were their ages, which alone would have made if difficult. One of the boys was incontinent and that wasn't even easy for a mom and dad to deal with. As if that wasn't enough, to our knowledge, no one had any kind of training to assume the role of nurse's aide and that is what is needed. In truth, for a lot of what we are called on to do, there is no training. You improvise until you have it down right and learn by doing because you must.

The same conclusions apply to the other two obvious classes of potential caregivers: friends and family members.

They say that the average persons of the ages of my wife and myself can count true friends on the fingers of one hand—and feel fortunate to do so. At this point, that dwindles down to maybe two or three. After a tour of duty or two, there might well be a lasting stress on the friendship, for the simple reason that it is NOT EASY! It isn't wise to involve friends.

That leaves family members. Unless you have them living in the same general area as you do, that fact alone eliminated most of them. Should you be fortunate enough to have some that live nearby, you still have to consider (1) their ages, (2) physical condition, and (3) training (or more probably, lack of it). After considering all of these obvious drawbacks to getting help from anyone or any group other than yourselves, you roll up your sleeves and keep on doing what you have been doing, whenever the aides depart or when they don't show up at all.

As an example, so help me, while I'm writing this, we find ourselves without a home health aide for the 7:30 AM—12:30 PM shift today. A new aide had been assigned by the agency. One aide, who had been here for the past several days, kept picking things up, asking personal questions such as, "How much did this cost? Where did you get this"? Jane called the agency and told them that her conduct was improper and out of line. They agreed and said they would talk to the lady. They did, but when she returned here, she was visibly upset and wound up walking out. Jane again called the agency and the management person on duty advised her that she and I "rolled up our sleeves", pitched in, washed him, dressed him and got him onto his power lift chair. The aide's walking out took place while I was writing this chapter and it wasn't until I took a break, left the room where I'm working, that I discovered what had transpired.

My wife wore a smile, and so did Nicky. The aide had gotten on their nerves, we had put up with it several days longer then we should have and it finally resolved itself; we had had enough; we complained; we concluded that she might walk out or get her nose out of joint. She did both. But we were better off without her than we were with her being here, though we wound up having no help for that morning. The agency promises a replacement, which might not be any better.

A final word about caregiving that has helped me many times when things pile up. I'm tired, irritable, or the patient seems unduly demanding. Maybe, for the night, suddenly, no one is coming to help. Don't take it out on the patient, your wife or even the cat. Tell yourself that this is the price you must pay to honor your commitment to your loved one to keep him or her in your home and out of an institution as long as there is breath left in you!

CHAPTER EIGHT

Two Resources For NEURO-FIBROMA-TOSIS—
Plus Over Twenty Toll-Free Health Info Numbers
For a Variety of Major Health Conditions
Of Diseases You May Encounter

ALSO: Valuable Insights on Obtaining Services for Your
Loved One

One of the most difficult, most frustrating, but also the most important task you will find yourself struggling with, is obtaining services for your loved one.

The fact that the bulk of our efforts in obtaining services involved primarily our identical twin sons would lead you to assume that the approval of services for them would also be identical. In the majority of instances, this was true, but there were times when one son would be approved for something and the other son denied.

A case in point was Medicaid prescriptions. While Bobby lived, both boys had Medicaid cards calling for co-payment for their Medicaid for their Medicaid drugs. Suddenly, Nicky's card bore the notation "Exempt from Co-Pay". Bobby's did not say this, so we had to continue paying a small co-payment for his medications. Little money was involved, but we were curious why one boy became exempt and the other not. We decided not to pursue the matter, reasoning that there was always the likelihood that, instead of making Bobby's card exempt from co-pay, they could well decide to take Nicky's exemption away. Other instances involved similar inconsistencies.

For the purpose of this chapter, "services" mean benefits or a program funded by one of the following:

SOCIAL SECURITY   MEDICAID   STATE AGENCY
NON-PROFIT AGENCIES   PRIVATE INSURANCE

State Agency—such as, in many states, Department of Mental Retardation (in South Carolina, known as the South Carolina Department of Disabilities and Special Needs) with a greatly expanded agenda and mandate.

Private Insurance—usually through a group, due to employment or part of a retirement benefit. Or could be health insurance purchased on an individual (or family) basis.

During the thirty-nine years since our twins were born, we have had extensive experience in trying to obtain services for them from most of the above listed sources. In many cases, it took considerable time and effort merely to identify *which* one of the groups listed above had the answer to our search.

One of the basic facts we learned was that, more often than not, things seldom seemed to come together for a favorable ruling the first time around.

Another conclusion follows the first one. You can't afford to give up, but you need to keep trying, as often as two, three or even more times if necessary to receive approval for the services you're seeking, or to press for clarification of anything you don't understand.

Timing is most important and since you have no way of knowing or anticipating exactly what time you should make your applications or appeals, it is all the more reason to make consistent, repeated attempts. This way, you increase your chances of hitting at the opportune time.

SUPPLEMENTAL SECURITY INCOME (SSI)

Sometime in 1984, both Bobby and Nicky were found eligible for SSI by the Social Security Administration. This made them also eligible for medical assistance from the Pennsylvania Department of Welfare. From that date on, there began a chaotic outpouring of computer generated letters from the Social Security Administration. The intent of the letters was to inform us that, for reasons never understood by us, the boys' checks were to stop and we were directed to refund to the government money already sent to them. Of course, we complied. I have a copy of a letter I sent to the manager of the Social Security office in York, pleading for an explanation of the confusing directions.

Being approved for SSI also meant that the boys were eligible for Medicaid and that Medicaid would pay for their Medicaid health insurance premiums. That is why it is so important to have them qualified for SSI and to remain so. But when they were taken off (sometimes only two or three months after again being certified as eligible), we never understood why and could never find anyone that was able to explain it.

After we moved to Summerville, South Carolina in April of 1988, the boys were ruled eligible by the North Charleston, South Carolina office of the Social Security Administration. Nevertheless, we received a Medicare notice dated October 13, 1988, terminating Bobby from SSI, requesting a refund, while Nicky, his identical twin received no such notice.

By then I had all I could take and decided, win, lose, or draw, to get to the bottom of it. I got the name of the manager of the downtown Charleston, South Carolina office of Social Security and, as Representative Payee for the boys, wrote a forceful, but polite letter, outlining the never-ending inconsistency and the confusing "on-again off-again" directives. In effect, I asked that the situation be stabilized and that they both be declared SSI/Medicaid eligible or explain why not, especially since they were yet again, recently ruled eligible by a SSA office. No one's circumstances had changed in the interim and there-fore, nothing that we were aware of had taken place to cause a reversal.

A representative of the North Charleston manager called me, took new applications over the phone for both Bobby and Nicky, and indi-cated that our situation would be resolved. In fact, there were no further contradictory reversals and the boys have remained eligible ever since.

Effective December 1984, Bobby was awarded Social Security bene-fits for disability based on my earnings record. Nicky's award was effec-tive October 1, 1985. They still continued to get SSI monthly checks, but for reduced amounts.

SOCIAL SECURITY

Applications for Social Security child's benefits were made on April 30, 1981. Applications for SSI were filed May 5, 1981. Their applications were disapproved June 22, 1981. A request for reconsideration was filed August 12, 1981. A request for a hearing was dated December 30, 1981.

The hearing was set for July 23, 1982. It was to be conducted by an Administrative Law Judge in Harrisburg, Pennsylvania (about 25 miles from our home in York). Prior to the hearing, I contacted an attorney in York whom I had previously met in the course of business. He professed to have expertise with Social Security disability appeal hearings and agreed to represent us for a fixed fee. At the last minute, just before the hearing was to commence, he waved a form in front of me to sign, changing the method of compensation to him from a fixed fee to a 25% contingency fee, stating it would be better for us. He was going for one-fourth of at least a year's worth of back benefits for both sons.

We thought he performed very poorly during the hearing, not allow-ing the boys to express themselves on any subject. He showed no signs of expertise with Social Security appeals procedures. The ruling by the judge was against the boys and their appeal was rejected.

One of the considerations held against Bobby and Nicky by the judge was the fact that both had participated in a government program known as "CETA". This was a make work type of operations that was designed to provide free lunches and recreation to inner-city youths and the elderly. The boys worked about two hours per day, five days a week. They served lunch and cleared tables. Even though no one operating a private business of this type would have hired them to do the tasks they were assigned to do and pay them for it, the fact that they could do it at all was held against them.

When we got down to street level, our attorney came over and stopped to talk to us as we were getting in our car. He turned to Nicky, who was leaning against a parked car for support and remarked, "It's okay, you can stop acting now, it's over". We were stunned!

As if to prove that I hadn't learned anything, I still felt that we needed an experienced person on our side, someone who actually had Social Security disability experience, especially on appeals. Although Social Security can turn you down, they also encourage and urge you to file an appeal. Results of these appeal hearings, or re-applications, show a high percentage of success on the second or even third time around.

I called the York County Bar Association and told them the kind of attorney we were looking for. They gave me the names of three attorneys who had gone on record with the Bar Association as having expertise in the field of practice desired. I picked out a name at random and made an appointment for the usual thirty-minute free consultation. That was the only face to face meeting with this attorney that I ever had.

After a month or so had elapsed with no word, I called the attorney's office, maybe three times over the second month. He offered no sign of progress, so I asked for the file of papers I had turned over to him to be returned to me. The attorney's response to my request was to send me a bill, listing several charges for meetings never taking place, amounting to several hundred dollars. He further advised me that, unless his bill was paid, he would not return my papers.

I promptly contacted the York County Bar Association Grievance Committee and filed a complaint. A date was set for a hearing at which the attorney and myself were to be present. The day before the hearing, the attorney's office called and told me that I could come and pick up the papers. The day after the hearing date, the Bar Association office called me and wanted to know why I didn't show up for the hearing. I explained that I had gotten my papers back and therefore had no further interest in pursuing the matter.

As the twins' physical condition worsened, we decided to go ahead by ourselves and re-apply for Social Security Disability benefits for them both. After the experience with the two attorneys, we concluded that we couldn't do much worse, so decided to proceed on our own.

Bobby's award came in December 1984, back dated to November of 1983. There is not doubt that the series of operations and hospitalization that he went through, starting in May of 1984 and ending in July of 1984, gave disability examiners solid evidence from Children's Hospital of Philadelphia records that would justify, once and for all, a finding of permanent and total disability. He was already well on his way to becoming a paraplegic, needing assistance with *every* daily living activity and in unrelenting pain. He had already lived, at the age of twenty-two, a year more than predicted.

Nicky's situation was also a matter of timing. His award was dated October 1, 1985. Sometime in the fall of 1985, I received a call from the disability claims office in Harrisburg, Pennsylvania, stating that they were awaiting a report from The Children's Hospital of Philadelphia regarding Nicky's condition. They told me that they could only wait a little longer to get it or they would have to close the file. I immediately called CHOP and pleaded with them to please send the report, explaining that a ruling on Nicky's Social Security application depended on it. Within the week, another call came from Harrisburg telling me that they had received the report and "everything had fallen into place". I felt if safe to conclude from that statement, that he would be approved for benefits.

Actually, it appears that several factors were involved in obtaining the favorable decision. One of them, of course, was his major surgery operation at CHOP in 1985. Another was the finding from his joint examination—with Bobby—at the Hershey Medical Center in 1982.

In addition, he was examined, specifically in connection with this application, by a neurosurgeon in Lancaster, Pennsylvania. Before the doctor began his examination, I asked him for a few minutes to explain to him exactly what Nicky's condition was and that Nicky positively was *not* acting or faking. I really believe that the doctor, by listening intently to me, did accept what I had to say and this well could have been a turning point for Nicky.

STATE AGENCY SERVICES

The following account probably does not represent a typical experience in trying to obtain services from a state agency. For one thing, it extended over a very long period of time; it involved a big dose of good fortune, opportune timing, and a lot of perseverance. Further, there was finally a resolution, in our favor.

No state agency wants to acknowledge the possibility that their rulings or decisions can be challenged. The reason is obvious: seldom does enough money exist to fund all of the requests and demands made upon them. On the other hand, they are bound to respond to appeals that are clearly outlined, courteously worded, directed to the right person, and based on a strong conviction that the position taken is right and just. Further, that it is truthful as to facts and complies with the agency's own guidelines as to what is required.

To give an idea of the full span of time it took to get a resolution of our efforts to obtain services from the South Carolina Department of Mental Retardation, that started in May of 1989 and ended March 10, 1994. Our original goal was to obtain respite care, since taking care of the boys was beginning to tell on us. We had some home health care (about two hours a day and four hours on Saturday) through South Carolina Community Long Term Care, a Medicaid program.

Originally, we were referred to the Dorchester County Board of Mental Retardation, an agency operating under what was then known as the South Carolina Department of Mental Retardation.

The boys were referred, by the County Board, for evaluation to the Coastal Region Community Programs Psychology Services. The testing was done at a Community Center in Ridgeville, South Carolina, a small community about ten miles from Summerville, our home. Administering the evaluation was Dr. Lester A. Finuf, Ph.D., Psychologist with the South Carolina Department of Mental Retardation.

I sat with Nicky and after that, Jane sat with Bobby. Dr. Finuf was very professional and tried to put the boys at ease and thus bring out the best in them. He did not patronize or talk down to them, so being fearful during the testing was not an excuse for below par results by the boys. I maintained contact with Dr. Finuf after the testing. At the conclusion of the questioning, he told me that he did not ordinarily test young persons whose conduct and responses were like those given by Bobby and Nicky. We were proud of them and felt that they had done their best, which we found always to be the case.

Results of the evaluation were, as one might expect, identical in just about all respects. Both boys were found ineligible for services because, "They score above the range of retardation in intelligence". Their adaptive behavior "composite score falls within the mild range of mental retardation". This was attributed by Dr. Finuf, primarily to their deficiencies in domestic skills.

Pointing out few facilities in South Carolina for persons such as Bobby and Nicky, Dr. Finuf felt that both boys ought to be separated from family care and that we needed to look to several agencies in Georgia that offered programs to persons with orthopedic problems but of normal intelligence. Needless to say, I contacted the referrals immediately, only to be told that the boys were not acceptable because they couldn't take care of themselves.

A Staffing and Certification Report was issued September 8, 1989, about six months after the evaluation/testing in May. It was signed by a Department of Mental Retardation psychologist—Director of D & E Services and a medical doctor who was assigned at the Coastal Center, a large facility near Summerville with housing for the more severely retarded.

This report followed closely the findings of Dr. Finuf's testing, i.e., not eligible for DMR services because neither son was considered mentally retarded. The same recommendations were made that we consider facilities in Georgia (which we had already checked out) and also that we contact the South Carolina Department of Vocational Rehabilitation, which we elected not to check out. The reason for our inaction was because, before leaving Pennsylvania, both boys were registered with the Pennsylvania Department of Vocational Rehabilitation and after several months under the York County branch, we could see no progress and withdrew from the program. They also were briefly enrolled in a computer training program in York, but funding could not be obtained.

I have often been asked (and have even asked myself) why we did not appeal the South Carolina DMR turndown in 1989. Very simply, because in my heart of hearts, I was confident that our sons were not retarded. I felt that I knew the boys and what they were capable of and therefore agreed with and accepted the findings of no mental retardation (other than mild).

Several years went by and in 1991, an entirely new (revised) program was announced. The South Carolina legislature had passed into law a revised State Code, agenda, and mission for what had been known as the SC Department of Mental Retardation. It would now be known as The South Carolina Department of Disabilities and Special Needs. The major difference in the revised program was that the applicant no longer had to be mentally retarded in order to qualify for services. Dr.

Finuf called to make me aware of this new initiative as being something that I might wish to look into.

I met with Dr. Finuf and on April 4, 1991, a Memorandum was sent by him, on South Carolina DMR letterhead (Coastal Regional Office, Summerville, SC), requesting reconsideration of the September, 1989 rulings of ineligibility. Updated medical reports were enclosed and the request was made pursuant to the related conditions proviso, a part of the "new" DMR.

On April 25, 199, a ruling came down from the central office level in Columbia, South Carolina, declaring that Nicholas Weeber was not eligible for DMR services through the powers outlined in 501-01-DD (this was the revised State code). No reason was cited for the declination. No mention was made of Robert Vincent Weeber (twin brother of Nicholas). I didn't have a copy of this April 25, 1991 letter until 1994.

Desperate for more services than we were getting through South Carolina Community Long Term Care Services, (a Medicaid program), I again approached Dr. Finuf in December, 1993, shortly before Christmas.

I asked Dr. Finuf why there had never been a ruling issued regarding Bobby's request for reconsideration in 1991. He did not offer an explanation. We discussed the specific reasons why services for Nicholas had been denied in April of 1991. Not fully understanding his explanation, I wrote him a letter on December 27, 1993 and he replied on January 6, 1994. My reaction was that his response did not address the issues I had raised and so stated.

While talking to Dr. Finuf shortly before Christmas, 1993, I expressed my frustration with the process. I was given a copy of a Memorandum written on August 20, 1993, on SCDMR letterhead, by a DMR central staff member in Columbia. The subject was: "Summary of Eligibility Criteria for DSN (Disabilities and Special Needs) and Related Issues".

Two groups or divisions of service were outlined. Group A, Mental Retardation and Related Disabilities, and Group B, Head and Spinal Cord.

After I had given this document extensive study, it seemed clear to me that, while Spinal Cord (Group B) Injury was a possibility for Nicky (since he had uncountable tumors, clusters of which were on or near his spinal cord), it appeared that Nicky (Bobby had passed away April 3, 1993), met every one of the four criteria listed under "Related Disabilities" and also met the definitions in connection with the 1991 request for reconsideration that my immediate reaction was "If my sons were not eligible, following the agency's own outline and definitions, then who is"? I reiterated this position at every opportunity, determined to get an answer, or a favorable ruling.

Not trusting my conclusion as to the criteria (since it seemed so clear cut). I discussed my interpretation with three professionals, familiar with our situation, whose judgment I respected. They unanimously agreed with me.

One of those was South Carolina Family Court Judge William J. Wylie, Jr. I kept Judge Wylie up to date on my efforts. I told him I was convinced that I somehow needed to talk directly with top management of the SCDDSN in Columbia. I wanted to go on record with them, with my belief that both boys had been eligible in 1991 according to their own guidelines, and that *Nicky was eligible now!* If my premise was correct, we should have a better than average case for back benefits on behalf of Bobby, going back to April of 1991 and surely should have led to Nicky's immediate eligibility.

Everyone needs a little luck. Or, as they say in the South, "Even a blind hog finds an acorn now and then".

Judge Wylie said he'd see what he could do. He had a classmate when in Law School at the University of South Carolina in Columbia, SC. He now believed she was working in the legal department of the SCDDSN in Columbia. He called her and as luck would have it (or was it an instrument of His intervention)? She was out of the office. The call was noted by the General Counsel, who returned the call to Judge Wylie to see if he could help.

Judge Wylie explained the situation and suggested that it would be helpful if I could call the General Counsel and explain my feelings about our case, with a request that they consider re-opening the file on Nicky (and I would not press for back benefits on Bobby's behalf).

Several weeks of phone calls followed, as well as a few letters back and forth between myself and the General Counsel. He was a gentleman throughout and listened attentively. I made every effort to conduct myself in a pleasant, but professional manner, while holding firm to my conviction that an injustice had been done to our sons by reason of the second turn down in 1991. I suggested that, for some reason, it did not appear that the department had all of the facts and a true picture of the boys' condition, as it related to their own guidelines. Also mentioned was the fact that, in April of 1991, it was a new program. I was sent a copy of the revised State Code on January 25, 1994 as it pertained to the DMR. This copy explained the mandated restructuring legislation revising the former Department of Mental Retardation's State Code. In turn, I sent a copy of the Memorandum I had been given by Dr. Finuf, announcing the new program, to the General Counsel, after he advised me that they were unable to locate the Memorandum in their office.

I had written on January 18, 1994, bringing up some issues about which I was unclear, and requesting that Nicky be reevaluated. The reply came back on January 25th, stating that my request was granted.

On Friday, February 18th, a licensed clinical psychologist came to the house and questioned Nicky. His written report was generally favorable and concluded by recommending Nicky for services, citing several reasons for his conclusion, the most important one being that Nicky appeared to require treatment similar to that administered to persons with mental retardation.

On March 10, 1994, a copy of a letter addressed to the Regional Director of the Coastal Region and signed by the Director of Admissions, (who took part in some of the conversations between myself and the General Counsel) was sent to us, advising that Nicholas Weeber "is appropriate for services at this time".

On April 22nd, we wrote a letter to the Admissions Director, expressing the appreciation of all of us for the granting of services. Our cases coordinator, Pam Furman, has worked diligently to make our program function and we express our gratitude also to Dr. Finuf for his assistance. And, we will never stop thanking Judge Wylie for his willingness to "open the door", thus giving me the opportunity to discuss my feelings about services to persons who had the authority to do something about it.

If you have faith in your cause, that it is necessary and just, you have to keep stating your case and trust that eventually it will come to the attention of the right person, who will listen. A plea to the Almighty for guidance won't hurt a bit!

In conclusion, I would be remiss if I didn't call your attention to a manual, published by the South Carolina Department of Disabilities and Special Needs, updated yearly, I believe. It is entitled, "A Practical Guide to Services".

There are ninety-six pages of helpful information about services and support groups for people with autism, head or spinal cord injuries, mental retardation, and related disabilities. It is also a reference for chambers of commerce, physicians, public schools, public libraries, government agencies, and other organizations that help people with disabilities and special needs find services in their local communities.

Of special interest to us in our quest for services was an agency listed as one offering advocacy services, including assistance to those who have been illegally denied a needed service by an agency or program. It is the South Carolina Protection and Advocacy System for the

Handicapped, Inc. (SCP&A). There are offices in four major South Carolina cities, including one in Charleston.

At one point, anticipating a possible further rejection of our attempts to obtain services from the DMR/DDSN, we contacted the SCP&A local office in Charleston. We talked to the attorney/manager, who advised that we needed to wait on a final decision before they could step in. Fortunately, we did not need to resort to this organization, as our case was resolved.

Although my knowledge of this resource is limited to its being in South Carolina, if living in another state, seek out such an agency there.

NEURO-FIBROMA-TOSIS RESOURCES

The following are the two major resources for those dealing with confirmed cases of neuro-fibroma-tosis (either NF 1 or NF 2) or those who are not certain whether they (or someone close to them) have the disease or not:

THE NATIONAL NEUROFIBROMATOSIS FOUNDATION, INC.

95 Pine Street, 16th Floor
New York, NY 10005
1-800-323-7938
Peter Bellerman, President

NEUROFIBROMATOSIS, INC.
8855 Annapolis Road, Suite 110
Lanham, MD 20706-2924
1-800-942-6825
Mary Ann Wilson, Administrative Director

OTHER RESOURCES: AARP

AARP has many programs designed to help with problems related to health, disability, caregiving and long term care. Someone (either the patient or their caregiver) must be a member of AARP in order to take advantage of these programs. With the annual membership fee only $8.00 for a person and spouse, this should make it affordable for most individuals. Here are just a few of the programs:

Planning for Incapacity: A Self–Help Guide

Each individual guide is written for a specific state and contains legal forms that your state requires.

Caregiving

Information for those who take care of disabled relatives and friends, even those living a long distance away. Materials cover both the support service options for those who stay at home and housing alternatives in the community. INA Pathway for Caregivers' is excellent.

Special

One of 3 special initiatives, the program for people with disabilities works to raise awareness, influence change and empower individuals to make a difference in their lives and the lives of others.

For more information about any of the above, or other AARP programs, call AARP's toll-free general inquiry number:

1-800-424-3410

(If not a member, you can inquire about joining.)

ADDITIONAL RESOURCES

For help to parents in working with teachers to develop your child's Individual Education Plan (IEP):

THE NATIONAL INFORMATION CENTER FOR CHILDREN
AND
YOUTH WITH DISABILITIES (NICHY)
P.O. Box 1492
Washington, DC 20013-1492
1-800-695-0285

For help with training and meaningful employment of persons with disabilities:

THE PRESIDENT'S COMMITTEE ON THE EMPLOYMENT OF
PERSONS WITH DISABILITIES
1331 F St., N.W.
Washington, DC 20004
(202) 376-6200

For names of attorneys specializing in Social Security cases in your state:

THE NATIONAL ORGANIZATION OF SOCIAL SECURITY
CLAIMANTS
AND REPRESENTATIVES
6 Prospect Street
Midland Park, NJ 07432
1-800-431-2804

TOLL-FREE HEALTH INFO NUMBERS
(Updated 7/24/01)

The following are toll-free numbers for health information resources for a number of widely experienced health conditions or diseases:

- Alzheimer's Association   1-800-272-3900
- American Diabetes Association   1-800-232-3472
- American Heart Association/Stroke Connection   1-800-242-8721
- Arthritis Foundation Information Hotline   1-800-283-7800
- Asthma and Allergy Foundation of America   1-800-727-8462
- Cancer Information Services   1-800-422-8237
- Dial Hearing and Screening Test   1-800-222-3277
- Grief Recovery Help-line   1-800-445-4808
- Lupus Foundation of America   1-800-558-0121
- National Headache Foundation   1-800-843-2256
- Brain Injury Association, Family Help-line   1-800-444-6443
- National Institute on Aging, Information Center   1-800-222-2225
- National Kidney Foundation   1-800-622-9010

Two Resources For NEURO-FIBROMA-TOSIS –Plus Over Twenty Toll-Free Health Info Numbers For a Variety of Major Health Conditions Of

- National Marrow Donor Program   1-800-573-6667
- National Mental Health Association   1-800-969-6642
- National Multiple Sclerosis Society   1-800-344-4867
- PMS Access   1-800-222-4767
- National Alliance of Breast Cancer Organizations   1-800-806-2226

To obtain a copy of "A Practical Guide to Services", the address is:

South Carolina Department of Disabilities & Special Needs,
Community Education Office
Post Office Box 4706
Columbia, South Carolina 29240
803-898-9600

WHAT WE LEARNED ABOUT OBTAINING SERVICES

In retrospect, we realize that almost every application that we have made for benefits on behalf of our sons was denied the first time around, most more than once.

For example, Social Security: an application, a denial; an appeal, a denial; the third time around, finally, an award of benefits. Elapsed time—over two years.

Medicaid: On and off again approval and then denial of benefits over a three-year period. Finally, a personal attention letter to the local agency manager, asking politely for a resolution of the matter, resulted in just that.

The South Carolina Department of Mental Retardation (later became The South Carolina Department of Disabilities & Special Needs): 1998, application, denial; 1991, application, denial; 1993, appeal to reopen the case, granted…benefits then awarded. Five years!

The best advice we can offer is to follow the Three Ps:

POLITE—Always be polite.

PERSISTENT—Make sure your case is just; if in doubt, find an advocate to confirm your belief.

PATIENCE—Doesn't mean waiting for long periods for nothing to happen, but be reasonable.

CHAPTER NINE

Nursing Homes—-Some Conclusions

Our first experience with nursing homes was when Bobby was admitted to a Low Country nursing home. This is detailed in Chapter Three, "The Medical Merry-Go-Round". To look at both the exterior and interior of this facility, you would never suspect the unsatisfactory conditions that existed within—and when told, most persons came close to not believing that it was true! At the time, this home was considered "state-of-the-art" and we felt fortunate that Bobby was admitted there. A local television station, WCBD Channel Two, aired segments on two consecutive evenings detailing the sad state of affairs at this nursing home, so our assessment of the situation was confirmed to the general public through these telecasts. I wrote to the out of state nursing home management company stating that his treatment was so bad that I felt Bobby was entitled to some kind of compensation for what he had been put through. I never had the courtesy of a reply.

As with most nursing homes, they had a "Bill of Rights" that each patient is entitled to. In Bobby's case, in this nursing home, it was only rhetoric.

Further, if a patient, or his representative, has to complain about too many of these items not being adhered to, then a management problem exists. What we were not aware of while all of Bobby's mistreatment was going on was that there was a South Carolina Nursing Home Advocate. At that time, it was a man and after Bobby was discharged, I called him to report what had been taking place. His territory was from Hilton Head Island (which is near the Georgia border) to Myrtle Beach (close to the North Carolina border). He explained that he could only be effective if the patient was still a resident of the home. Since then, I've been advised that this type of advocacy is now handled out of an office in Columbia, South Carolina (state headquarters for most state agencies). I honestly felt that this nursing home was very close to violating Bobby's civil rights, but we had so many other concerns, as always, that we opted to put the whole issue on hold.

When one of Charleston's major hospitals announced plans to construct a nursing home in a suburban location, I immediately called the hospital, spoke to a management lady regarding the project and requested that both of our sons be put on a potential resident list and that I expected that we would be either number one of two. At that time, an opening was several years away. Since Bobby was living then, my wish was, if they had to go to a nursing home and/or leave our household, that they be together. The hospital promised that, if they got an allotment of Medicaid beds from the State of South Carolina, their nursing home management company in Nashville, TN would let me know.

I kept checking back, but no word of any Medicaid beds. Finally the home opened, but we heard nothing further until one day the Admissions Director called and said they were updating their "list" of potential residents and wanted to know if we still wanted our sons' names on their list. We explained that Bobby passed away, but still wanted Nicky on the list.

Jane and I went to the home and were given a tour of the facility. This was now truly the most "state-of-the-art" nursing home in the Low Country. Because of my very early efforts, I assumed that, by this time, Nicky should be at the very top of the list, or close to it. It is hard to believe, but every time I visited to speak with the Admissions Director, before I could open my mouth to say a word, she would inform me that there had been no turnover of Medicaid beds and no indication that any beds were about to be vacated. For all I know, Nicky may still be on the "list".

Medicaid beds for young males are scarce as hen's teeth. If young males are articulate, well spoken, intelligent, etc., they are not going to be high on the list. They will require too much service. As far as official admission policy that nursing homes are to follow, there is literally none. They have only two requirements (for Medicaid patients). They must agree to accept the amount of reimbursement that is available and they must provide the Medicaid patient the same degree of service that the Medicare or private-pay residents receive. Other than that, they are free to admit or not admit. All they have to say is that the do not feel they can provide the level of service that your loved one appears to require, and that's it. Period!

Once admitted, you are protected against almost every conceivable situation that could take place in a nursing home. I called the Governor's Office in Columbia, South Carolina, inquiring for as much information as I could get in writing concerning exactly what nursing homes in the state were allowed to do and what they could not do. I was sent a manual that must have been three inches thick and if anything else can happen to a patient in a nursing home that isn't in this manual, no one needs to know about it. It is the most complete, thorough document I have ever read, and while I certainly didn't read every line, I read enough to convince me that the organization distributing the manual had apparently covered the field.

And who is this outfit? The National Citizen's Coalition for *Nursing Home Reform*. NCCNHR is a national, non-profit membership organization, founded in 1975, to improve the long-term care system and the quality of life for nursing home residents. This came about as a result of nursing home abuses that were so widespread and flagrant that the situation cried out for reform and/or regulation. In 1996, as a part of the Republican program, there was an attempt by the nursing home lobby to drop these "Survey Procedures", which are detailed instructions as to how to investigate complaints for everything you can think of regarding patient's treatment and/or patient's rights—the very existence of which has made life bearable for all nursing home residents. These safeguards were viewed by the nursing home lobby as too restrictive. I shuddered when I first learned of what they were planning to do, but believe their plan was eventually discarded. If you want a copy, either phone (703) 487-4600, or write:

National Technical Information Service

U.S. Department of Commerce

5285 Port Royal Road

Springfield, Virginia 22161

Sometime in 1995, an area nursing home, relatively new in the Low Country (and another "state-of-the-art" facility), called us concerning Nicky. They said that they had just been awarded an allotment of Medicaid beds and had gotten Nicky's name from Dorchester County Social Services as a person who was Medicaid eligible and ready to go into a Medicaid bed. We visited the home and were given the grand tour. It looked great and was not very far from where we live. As a result of our visit, two of the management staff came to our house; they interviewed Nicky, but to a far greater degree, my wife and I, also. We gave candid, truthful answers to their questions. When they left, the Christmas holidays were just around the corner, so we were told not to expect any decision until after the first of the year.

In the meantime, we agonized over the prospect of actually putting Nicky in a nursing home, even in what seemed to be a decent and modern environment. Finally, since so many of our friends and our minister felt it was a step we'd eventually have to take, we better not pass this up, as it might not come around again, and certainly not when we would need it the most. In addition to the hurt it would do to Nicky, we would lose his Social Security and SSI as approximate $5,000 a year. Since we had recently lost Bobby's Social Security through his death, that would be another devastating blow to our economy and would pose bad consequences for us. Still, we felt that we should grab this opportunity never telling Nicky in order not to upset him.

After the first of the year, I contacted the Admissions Director and apparently the Medicaid bed was up for grabs. At the last minute, a call came, informing us that, "I had to give his (Nicky's) bed to a man coming out of a hospital bed". I ran into the Admissions Director later at a Health Fair and she advised me that Nicky didn't get the bed "because you and your wife weren't ready to give him up"! Those were her words and confirmed what I had been told, i.e., if you want to get someone into a Medicaid bed in a nursing home, have them admitted to a hospital. Then, the theory is that the hospital will—at probably an early point—want to push them out and presumably put pressure on the nursing home to admit them with the appeal that there is no where else to go with the person.

Another suggestion (what can you lose?), is to visit a nursing home, speak to the Admissions Director, and ask what their policy is. Do they have a list? They'll probably tell you how many are ahead of you. Then ask if there is an flexibility on their part in working with someone who faces a critical, emergency situation if their loved one is not admitted to a Medicaid bed. I had one such Director tell me that she was flexible and tried hard to take care of such emergency situations, *if* they came at a time when they had or were about to have a vacancy, and obviously that is not always the case, although it may well be. I think these methods hold out more promise than going to half a dozen nursing homes and getting on each "waiting list". In almost every case, you will wind up waiting!

And now, so that you will be able to see and read a nursing home's typical "Resident Bill of Rights", one is reprinted here:

"PATIENT/RESIDENT BILL OF RIGHTS"

Every patient has the right:

To considerate and respectful care

To know what kind of care and treatment will be given

To refuse medication and treatment

To be free from mental and physical abuse

Freedom to voice a complaint

To be heard and receive a reasonable response

Not to fear punishment for an action

To actively participate in the plan of care unless medically contra-indicated

To expect reasonable continuity of that care

To be informed of and know about their medical condition unless medically contra-indicated

To expect continued treatment of identified medical or psycho-social problems, and monitoring to prevent and detect possible new problems

To respect and privacy as it relates to their medical care progress

To have every reasonable allowance for individuality in recreational activities

To religious observance of their choice

To attend group activities or to decide not to attend, if they prefer

To maintain contacts in the community

To the use of the telephone

To bring clothing and personal possessions with them

To handle personal funds, to delegate others to handle their funds, and receive appropriate accounting of what is spent on their behalf, if the health care facility is authorized to manage their funds

To occupy the same room with a spouse, if both are residents and if the physician permits

To be informed first before being transferred to another facility and why this is necessary

Not to be required to perform services for the facility unless there is a therapeutic purpose to such activity as part of the "plan of care"

SIGNATURE: _____

WHAT WE LEARNED FROM NURSING HOMES

Nursing homes can refuse admission (and do) to otherwise qualified applicants, by simply saying that they do not feel able to give such a person the service that he or she requires.

"Lists" that Admission Directors maintain (for future admissions) are just that—lists that are not written in stone. You (or your loved one) are probably not on any list, but most admission directors are willing to listen—your situation is a real emergency, for example, involving caregivers who absolutely can't carry on any more, some will make an effort to admit you. Even then, they have to have an immediate or pending vacancy at the time you need a bed there.

Regulations governing what goes on in a nursing home are very specific and generally adhered to by the management. However, don't count too much on DHEC or the State Ombudsman for nursing homes. If the problem is ongoing and the patient is still in the home, the Ombudsman should be able to intervene. If the patient has been discharged, they claim there's not much they can do.

Thirty percent of persons recently polled said they'd rather be dead than to be confined in a nursing home. This pretty much confirms what our remaining son has told us many times: "If you put me in a nursing home, my life is over."

A nursing home may be "state-of-the-art", with lovely furnishings, décor and good food, but if the place is understaffed, the workers overworked and underpaid, with an uncaring administration, life for the inmates will not be worth living.

Finally, look hard and don't be afraid to ask questions—lots of them. The bad nursing homes won't like it, but the good ones should welcome it.

CHAPTER TEN

Some Activities The Boys Enjoyed

Bobby and Nicky planned and did a lot of things together, although as Nicky confided after Bobby passed on, they didn't always agree on everything, but Nicky said that he went along nevertheless in order to keep peace. "Two Against the World" sounds maudlin, but if ever words described their general attitude, those words do. I can remember times walking into the room that they both shared during the day and having one or both politely but firmly ask me to leave, as what they were discussing was private. And Jane got pretty much the same treatment if she entered their room while a private discussion was underway. Even though what they were talking about might not qualify as privileged information to us, we tried to honor their requests and left their room at once.

Most persons, usually those who didn't know the twins well, have a preconceived idea that they were going to encounter two boys who would probably be sitting there, staring into space and not speaking or seeming to hear anything. When the reality (which was that they were both very personable, well spoken, with above-average vocabularies) sank in, many visitors or new home health aides were visibly taken aback. Watching their reactions, I could detect an air of disbelief and more than a slight touch of resentment. The boys just didn't fit the mold and I've always been grateful for that.

We got them an electric typewriter and they took turns using it. While one typed, the other would work out the various scenarios their imagination was creating. These were fantasy biographies; consisting of action adventures and featured their ministers, barber, and whoever else they could think of. Some of these went on forever and came in episodes, which they would send off and then pick up the story later for seemingly endless story lines.

Another activity that kept them busy was writing fan letters to television stars, mostly of the "soap" variety. They would write for autographed pictures and before they finally called a halt to this endeavor, they had a collection of approximately one thousand photos. Several of these TV personalities went on to become continuing correspondents, some on a regular basis. Kate Linder wrote faithfully. She and Melody Thomas-Scott, both of *The Young and Restless*, had been advised by mail that Bobby was terminal. About one hour after Jane and I returned from a local hospital, where Bobby was dead on arrival, Ms. Linder called to inquire about Bobby. Of course, we had to give her the sad news of his passing. Ms. Thomas-Scott wrote Nicky that he was her best "pen pal".

Nicky wrote to soap star Michael O'Leary, of *Guiding Light*, praising his performance. Mr. O'Leary was so impressed that he called long distance from New York City. He told me that he had just received Nicky's letter and it was the **nicest fan letter that he had ever received from anyone** and he had to talk to the person who wrote it! A couple of weeks later, Michael O'Leary called again and told me he had been thinking about a way whereby perhaps he and Nicky could get together. He said he had a very strong wish to meet Nicky and tentative plans were discussed. He was careful not to make an absolute promise as the arrangements would be difficult for both parties—his work obligations to the program and Nicky's limitations as to travel because of his physical condition. It hasn't happened yet, and Nicky despairs that it may never take place. However, he keeps writing, keeps watching for Michael on *Guiding Light*, and keeps hoping that eventually they will meet.

We are proud of both sons and the fact that they have come so far from what appeared to be a disastrous beginning. Certainly they both have come a very long way and Jane and I are happy to see Nicky carry on despite the loss of his best friend and identical twin. Incidentally, Nicky has never openly cried over Bobby's death, but we know that he misses him, as we all do.

Between them, they had assembled a better than average collection of videos, with a heavy selection of the original *Star Trek* episodes. While living in York, Pennsylvania, we took them both to several *Star Trek* conventions, where they got to meet (and get autographs on pictures of a number of the cast members). We used to drop them off at the Hunt Valley Maryland Marriott Hotel, see that they had lunch and left them to watch the program and after, get the autographs, and meet the stars. They were still mobile, though Bobby did need a cane. Because they were obviously handicapped, they usually were permitted to go to the head of the line, thus avoiding having to stand a long time. The boys would chat briefly with whoever was signing the pictures and were able to get a few laughs out of the cast members. Never at a loss for words, their gift of gab stood them in good stead during these meetings.

In 1980 or 1981, a year or so before the boys graduated from York Suburban High School with their "Special Education" diploma, they entered a program with a name similar to: Diversified Occupational Training. They elected to volunteer at York Hospital and were assigned duties as follows: Nicky went to the print shop and was kept busy collating papers. Bobby was assigned to a service called "Tel-Med". He sat at a switchboard, where people would call in, requesting that audio tapes be played, according to the subject they wanted, which choices were printed in the local York phone book. They would specify which tape they wanted to listen to, Bobby would pick the tape out of wherever it was filed, and put it in the player. Every now and then, a disturbed person would storm into the hospital lobby, where Bobby was stationed. Typically, the person was a religious fanatic and would start preaching or muttering words that were almost unintelligible. This would upset

Bobby. Also, people would call in and start arguing about their electric or telephone bills, regarding which the boys could do nothing.

After graduation, they continued. It kept them occupied, and when they finally resigned, each had volunteered a total of one thousand hours and were awarded pins confirming this accomplishment.

CHAPTER ELEVEN

Medical Equipment Providers

Through the years, we must have dealt with over a dozen medical equipment providers. For the most part, there have been few problems, with deliveries being made when needed and billings in accordance with the facts. Still, there is ample opportunity in the system for suppliers to take advantage and Medicare is the target for most of the excesses. No wonder Medicare is having problems! Yet, in many instances, the amounts they approve are astounding. In one case, an item was approved and billed to Medicare for $10,400. Some custom fitting was involved and two return visits had to be made by the supplier, after the initial delivery, to make adjustments. I have no way of knowing if this is true, but was told by a dealer that the identical item could be obtained by him for four thousand dollars. They probably weren't allowing anything for custom fitting, but even so, it seems like a large spread.

For many years, the boys had both Medicare and Medicaid, with the latter as the payor of last resort. In addition, we carried group health insurance on them (as well as ourselves) through Jane's employment and/or retirement benefits, which was considered secondary coverage. When we received Medicare's "Explanation of Benefits" forms regarding a claim we had filed, it would advise us that Medicare was sending a copy to Medicaid to see if additional benefits could be paid, either completely ignoring or not realizing the existence of secondary insurance that should have come before billing Medicaid. After Bobby died, we had Nicky insured with our group insurance, but the cost had gone to forty dollars a month. He could have had a Medicare supplement for a lot less money and we argued for this, but the insurer was adamant and would not budge. Since claims were seldom paid for the boys under their secondary insurance and because of the cost, we dropped that coverage on Nicky.

Another Medicare policy regarding equipment concerned the issue of equipment rental. Some items Medicare insisted be rented for a certain number of months, after which the patient was offered an opportunity, in writing, as to whether they wanted to continue renting the item or purchase it. The patient is advised that, if they continue renting the equipment, the supplier is entitled to bill them every six months for service/maintenance WHETHER IT IS NEEDED OR NOT OR WHETHER THE EQUIPMENT IS SERVICED OR NOT. It would certainly seem that a client would be foolish indeed to choose the continued renting option.

In one case, the supplier claimed I didn't return the signed form, so kept on billing Medicare for continued renting of the item. Medicare advised me that the supplier's billing was so fouled up that I could not exercise the purchase option, but would have to wait. This battle with the provider, Medicare, and me went on for over three years after delivery of the item, which was erroneously billed as a purchase when it should have been delivered on a rental basis, to begin with. It had optional extra equipment on it that I did not order. When questioned, the provider explained that the "add-ons" were the result of a model improvement. The billing was rendered using my Medicare number instead of the twin's number for whom the item was ordered. In fact, there were so many errors made in the entire transaction that even I would have great difficulty in putting down on paper the chronology of the whole ordeal.

Another medical equipment situation that I thought had been dealt with flared up again. It is another example of a provider ignoring the signed rental-purchase option (or claiming they never received it) and continuing to bill for rentals, including two six-month service/maintenance charges, each the equivalent of a month's rental charge. This was bad enough, but the billing continued long after the item had been picked up!

Finally, I called Medicare to report what was going on and they connected me to the "Anti-Fraud" unit, where I explained to the manager what was still going on, almost a full year after the item had been returned (the owner of the dealership had picked up the item personally and I had a copy of his signed receipt). I *never* alleged fraud, because I wasn't certain of the facts in the case. That is up to Medicare. They advised me later, by letter, that the matter was being dealt with and that the provider was being ordered to refund all charges made after the item had been returned. They thanked me for reporting it and said they intended to keep an eye on the provider. Low and behold, a few weeks later, I received a Medicare "Explanation of Benefits" form that indicated that the same provider had submitted an invoice for a maintenance charge earlier in the year. Medicare paid nothing. I called Medicare again and asked how this claim could even be considered and was asked to send them documentation of my report, which was done!

A recent incident indicates the complexity and cost of health care when you are caught in an emergency situation. Hurricane "Fran", one of 1996's more destructive hurricanes, was bearing down on the Charleston, South Carolina coastal area. We had been through "Hugo" and evacuated twice, once to avoid the storm, then, after returning home from Columbia, South Carolina to find no electricity and substantial damage to the house, leaving again to stay with relatives and friends in two nearby states. With "Fran", we had arranged to stay with our youngest daughter, Mary, who lives in the Atlanta Metro area, if it turned out that we really needed to evacuate.

Not wanting to take a chance with Nicky's well being, we left with the storm reported to be veering away, but only four hours from Charleston. We departed and when we got to our daughter's house, radio and TV reports made us realize that we could have stayed in Summerville! Now, we needed both a hospital bed and a portable commode for Nicky, so my daughter called a pharmacy specializing in health care equipment rental and ordered both items. Despite Nicky's Medicare and Medicaid coverage, the provider said that he could not honor either one. This was not unreasonable, since Nicky already had, on his record through Medicare, both a bed and a portable commode in our home in Summerville. We stayed two nights in Georgia and the rental bill was one hundred fifty-six dollars. The invoice indicated that this amount was for one month's rental, although the equipment was returned after two days. We would have been lost without it.

Medicare will only pay for the *mechanism* on a power lift chair. I thought that our secondary insurance would pick up the difference, but they denied payment on the grounds that they were obligated to follow Medicare's policy. Obviously, you can't sit on *just* the mechanism, so, even though Medicaid did pay some, we still had to pick up a sizeable portion of the cost, which suddenly went from four hundred fifty dollars to five hundred fifty dollars to "see what Medicare will do".

WHAT WE LEARNED FROM DEALING WITH MEDICAL HOME EQUIPMENT PROVIDERS

Even on the day that I write this copy, front page headlines in the local paper trumpet, "Medical fraud cases up." And the health care system has been easy to defraud. The rip-offs filter down from some for-profit hospitals to the independent medical equipment provider in your own neighborhood.

*We recently needed a "gait" belt (used to transfer patients that can't stand alone). A local provider quoted forty dollars—would have to order it from a supplier and would have taken at least a week to two weeks before we would have received it. I went to Wal-Mart's Pharmacy department, they called their regional warehouse, I had it the next day; cost—five dollars. We don't know whether Medicare would have approved forty dollars or not—and we don't know that they wouldn't. Anyway, I paid for it out of pocket, got it quicker, and saved **someone** money. I felt like I'd done a good thing.*

So, shop around. Use your phone and Yellow Pages. Chances are you can either save yourself money (if you're paying) or save money for Medicare, Medicaid, or your insurance company.

*A tip-off to a potential rip-off: when the owner or clerk says, "Let's see what Medicare will do" (as he adds another hundred dollars or so to an item that he could easily have billed **without** adding on another hundred dollars). Sadly, Medicare often does approve the higher price, but you can still be alert. Ask questions. And at least try to get the best price. If we all would do that, health care costs would begin to go down.*

*If you rent equipment from a provider through Medicare and return it, **get a dated receipt** and watch your Medicare billings. If the provider contin-ues to bill Medicare **after** you returned the item, **YOU need to notify Medicare**, otherwise, they have no way of knowing that you did return it. Let Medicare decide whether it is fraud, but whatever is going on is wrong!*

*Wheelchairs, lift devices and hospital beds are subject to rentals through Medicare. When given an option to purchase or continue rent-ing the equipment, **PURCHASE!***

CHAPTER TWELVE

The Present Reality

Looking for an answer that might give us a new perspective on the meaning of reality, I asked my wife one morning, "Please give me your definition of reality, as it pertains to our situation, in one sentence". Her answer took me aback momentarily; "Grim", she replied.

Expert writers are telling me that a writer needs to be able to describe their book in one sentence…but they didn't say that you had to do it in *one word*. I can't argue with her response, for there is the quality of grimness that pervades what we are faced with every twenty-four hours, week after week, month after month, and year after year. No single thing that we are called on to do, from minute to minute, is that demanding or physically or mentally exhausting, but the sum total finally takes its toll, like the proverbial drop of water "that weareth away a stone" or the Chinese "water torture cure".

Reality is the fact that neuro-fibroma-tosis is a progressive disease; it can never (so far) get better.

After the gene that causes NF-1 was identified several years ago, hope surfaced that gene therapy could be developed that would inhibit the further growth and development of tumors. The United States Army Medical Command has spent in excess of thirty-two million dollars over a five year period on NF research and their program continues. When I became aware of the program, I immediately made an effort to get Nicky enrolled in it, but after submitting MRI scans to one of the several neurosurgeons taking part in the effort, we were advised that his case was too far advanced to admit him into the program. He would have had to take a shot every day and that would not have been easy for him—or us—to undertake. One neurosurgeon, in the Washington, DC area, told me on the phone that, if one of Nicky's tumors turned cancerous, to contact him and he would see what could be done.

The reality is that I need to get up a little after 6 a.m. each and every morning and fix the medicine that Nicky will need. When Nicky calls me from his room at 6:45 a.m., I then call Jane to come and help and we both go into his room and perform about eight tasks, which takes about five minutes, reminiscent of a Chinese fire drill! We arrange his urinal to help him urinate while lying in his hospital bed, give him a small amount of orange juice to ease his dry mouth and throat. At 7:30 a.m., seven days a week, the home health aide is due to arrive and she takes over, to bathe and dress him and give him his breakfast, some of which has to be administered by her. If she does not arrive, either on time or at all, Jane then takes over and I assist her as she directs me. This is not an uncommon occurrence, so, when the phone rings around 7 a.m., we flinch a little and wait for the shoe to drop. A new aide can't come—for any one of a number of reasons we've heard many times before and now and then, a new reason that is often unique or ingenious. The three of us grumble, but pitch in and take care of his needs. I'm thankful that we're here for him and we both know that, as always, Nicky is appreciative of that and tells us so, often apologizing because he realizes that his condition is the root cause of it all. This scenario, repeated with great frequency, is part of what reality is.

At around 2:30 p.m., Jane and I again collaborate to give him a snack and a drink, then help him to use the portable commode. At 4:30 p.m., we sweat out the arrival—or non-arrival—of the aide for the 4:30—6:30 shift. If the aide shows, she gives him supper, gets him in his pajamas and with my help, into his hospital bed. The aide vacuums his room and hall area and then departs. I then bring him the two newspapers that he reads each evening along with his latest *Star Trek* novel and a few of the tabloids that he buys every week. Then Jane and I sit down to supper.

At 8:00 p.m., I bring him some medication along with a drink to take it with. I assist him in using the urinal in bed. At this point, if Jane looks as though she's awake, I can go to bed. If not, I also brush his teeth, set up his intercom in his bed, change his VCR tapes (that goes on all day and part of the night), and anything else he wants done that he can't do for himself.

At around 9:30 p.m., I get up fix some orange juice for Nicky, cat food for his cat, get the cat into his bedroom for the night, give him the orange juice, assist him in using the portable urinal, turn the lights off and go back to bed. He will usually call me in about an hour, to use the urinal again. After that, he is liable to call for help anywhere from midnight to 6:00 a.m. Whenever he calls—and no matter how often—I get up and help him. At a little after 6 a.m., I get up again to start the day's round of activities. That is the reality of a typical day, from day to day after day.

There is no way of knowing what Nicky's mortality rate is at this juncture. It was predicted that he would be lucky to make it past age twenty-one, but he's already lived eighteen years beyond that. Will he be here at age forty, to see the year 2002 and the next millennium, or even next week? The reality is that uncertainty will continue and truly the philosophy of "live each day" is apropos here.

There are many instances where persons who should be close to the boys or at least understanding of their condition, choose to distance themselves or ignore them completely. That kind of reaction is apparently a classic case of denial. They find the boys' predicament (and by extension, our predicament) more than they can handle. To avoid feeling guilty, they adopt an attitude of indifference and denial, even going to the extreme of blaming the boys and/or us, as their parents. Where there should be love, compassion, and concern, there is the opposite—resentment, condemnation, and rejection.

Bobby' death softened a few of the positions, but most of the hurtful attitudes continue unabated. When, in a moment of frustration, over the non-arrival of a scheduled home health aide, we voiced our dissatisfaction with the situation, we could hear voices telling us that "as long as you choose to keep Nicky at home (implied) and not in a nursing home (where he belongs), you have to accept the consequences (and don't complain)".

This said as if we had an overflowing basket of options, any one of which could be easily adopted and would immediately solve our problem, but none of which would consider Nicky's feelings.

One part of this attitude is true. It *is* our choice to maintain Nicky at home. There are emotional consequences that would devastate Nicky and ourselves were we to give up on our efforts and start proceedings for his admission to a nursing home This in addition to financial damage to our economy that would have profound ill effects. In reality, he would probably view it as us abandoning him.

Nicky's pain from his many tumors continues to get more intense. A pain doctor at MUSC's Pain Clinic has started him on a new medication and has rearranged the rest of his medications for maximum pain relief. He is now getting close to the kind and amount of pain medication that is often prescribed for terminal patients. The idea is to eliminate as much pain as possible, but not to create harmful side effects or drug dependency. There are some side effects, from time to time, but so far, there is no indication of drug dependency.

It is hard to account for much that has taken place. We have to accept the fact that, despite our human efforts, the final events will be dictated by His actions and we can expect that, as always, it will be for the best!

On January 22, 2001< Nicky finally entered a group residential home in a nearby Summerville, S.C. subdivision. I see him at least four times a week and we talk by phone daily. His care is basically good. The Dorchester County (SC.) Department of Disabilities & Special Needs staffs the home.

CHAPTER THIRTEEN

The Future

As the popular song of some years back advised us, "The Future's Not Ours To See". Undoubtedly just as well! Sometimes we have trouble seeing the tunnel, let alone the light that's supposed to be at the end. The disintegration of society is beyond our control, but we are the victims of it by the conduct of some who are sent to help Nicky. We don't see any dramatic change in the conditions that exist that have caused some person's value systems to not only go downhill, but to cease to exist.

A talk show host made this statement not too long ago; "Persons from different cultures either cannot co-exist for very long or at all". If ever any spoken words had profound meaning, these surely do. This truth is revealed here on not only a weekly basis, but almost daily. We have seen so many types of individuals and examples of mentalities (or lack of them) that I have often wondered if it would not be wise to replace our standard front door with a revolving type, at the same time making it easier on those who enter and also ourselves.

We have counseled Nicky, if pushed too far, to assert himself...not to be rude or arrogant, but to practice what, in an auto, would be termed "defensive driving". It is inevitable that he will be called upon to deal with others more and more on his own and better to start doing some of it now, than to wait until one or both of us are no longer around.

To the best of our ability and with both limited financial resources and ability to improve our financial picture, we have tried to provide a measure of economic and physical security for Nicky's future.

We have established a Living Trust, with Nicky's well being the paramount concern. This despite outspoken criticism that all but says, "What are you guys doing with a 'Living Trust'? The size of your estate, upon the deaths of both of you, is not nearly enough to justify such a trust, (unless you are both run over and killed in a common carrier accident)".

We've put every asset that we have into funding it and it certainly could use a substantial infusion of cash to be able to provide the *supplementary* financial aid to Nicky that could take care of some of his needs that otherwise might not be met. We have faith that He will find a way, regardless of whether we're around to know about it or not.

One thing that we have established is that the best arrangement that we could come up with is the designation and agreement for Nicky's younger sister, Mary, to act as his guardian and also his Successor Trustee of our Trust, succeeding us, upon the death of both of us. It is not a perfect choice, as Mary has heavy family and job responsibilities of her own. We know her to be a caring person who will conscientiously carry out her obligations under the Trust. The fact that she lives and works in the Atlanta area and Nicky is here in the South Carolina Low Country (and will probably have to remain here), with a well-established program of services and home health care makes it less than a perfect situation. With Mary's efforts and His intervention and support, Nicky will never be neglected or forgotten. We have to close our eyes and rest, knowing that we gave it our best shot, kept the faith, and stayed the course.

We can, at that point, look forward to being reunited with Bobby, our deceased parents, and all other loved ones. At peace with Thee.

The Many Legacies Of Bobby Weeber

When Bobby was only a few years old, his pediatrician told us that Bobby (and his twin brother Nicky) was retarded, and "you'll have to learn to live with it".....also, "you'll be fortunate if they live beyond age 21." Bobby proved him wrong on both counts. Nevertheless, when Bobby passed away Saturday afternoon, April 3, 1993, at 1:48 p.m., our entire family's reaction was one of disbelief, mine perhaps even more so. Although Bobby had been pronounced terminally ill on February 22 (on account of a usually benign tumor that had turned cancerous) and given 60 days to live, the reality of his death in the emergency room at Trident Regional Medical Center seemed final.

For a week afterward, the seeming unfairness and injustice of his life of suffering and death were almost unbearable. How could God do this—and more importantly, why? I was angry at God and told Him so. I had tried to assure Bobby that God had not singled him out to punish or destroy him, that He was not a vengeful God. But the alternative was: "if that is so, why is my number up—what have I done wrong? I've tried to be a good son." My constant answer was that God had a plan for him and would not desert him. For over 90 days, I had to tell Bobby almost daily as he cried out in pain, "I'm sorry, we're doing all that we know to do—there is nothing more except for all of us to pray for remission or divine intervention." But neither ever came.

In the final week preceding his death, I got more into Bobby's condition with him than I had before. I suggested to him that he not go out with anger or malice towards those who had maligned him or ill-treated him. I pointed out that would be inconsistent with the champion that he was. He gave me to understand that he agreed and forgave everyone. I should have done more of this and done it sooner, and if the situation arises again, no matter with whom, I will remember it. I finally realized that I couldn't bring Bobby back by crying and reproaching myself and that my focus had to shift to honoring his memory. What helped was an outpouring of praise and admiration for the character that he always displayed and the gallant battle he wage to live. Also, his coming to terms when he realized his death was inevitable. Two Presbyterian churches (in addition to his own, Summerville Presbyterian Church) recognized his passing. Countless cards, letters, phone calls and personal visits bore testimony to the fact that he was indeed a very special person.

Like Christ, Bobby was crucified. In suffering and dying, he touched many lives and by the way he handled it, caused some to reverse their attitudes of denial to ones of love and acceptance. Bobby gave new meaning to words like: "Courage, Love, Gratitude, Unselfishness, Grace, Devotion, Politeness, Humor, Creativity, Honesty" and many more. Little did he know that the legacies he left would help us to cope with his loss and put us on our mettle to live up to them. In the jargon of today, he is a hard act to follow. The real truth is that, as much as we loved him, cared for him and appreciated him for the person that he was, we realize that we didn't fully comprehend what we had. He has helped us find some meaning in his life and death. But in truth, he is not dead, but lives on in our hearts, lives and memory.

Bobby wanted so much to see "A Few Good Men" at the local theater, but we never made it. I like to think that God needed "a few good men" up there when he called Bobby's number. I'm not angry with God anymore—I hope He forgives me. He made the right decision—the suffering is over at last. And yes—if they can use a little humor where he has gone…an original joke, a pun or a gag…Bobby can deliver.

Nicky Weeber On TV!

Yes, it is true and I wanted my friends and correspondents to know about it! Actually, I'm only on the audio part of the 6 o'clock nightly "Live Five" news hour. Around 6:15, a segment called "Talkback" airs on WCSC, TV-5 in Charleston, SC. I call in and have been allowed to "get on" the program so much that a man who does accents claims he can mimic me to perfection simply by listening to me as I speak with the anchor!

It started some time back and got to the point I was invited to the TV studio in downtown Charleston to meet the anchors and watch the actual presentation of the news. I met the lead anchors…Bill Sharpe and Debi Chard; Charlies Hall, Weather and Warren Peper, Sports. Warren actually does the "Talkback" segment. There are others whom I have gotten to meet, such as Bill Walsh, Weather and other news reporters who serve as anchors on the weekend telecast.

I was invited back for a second visit and we went and took my current home health aide to help with loading and unloading me in and out of the car. I enjoyed it as much or more than the first visit. I have autographed pictures of most of the key persons. In the late afternoon, I often call in and ask to speak to one or more of the anchors. Sometimes I can talk to them and sometimes not if they are not in or busy.

I have followed the Simpson trial very closely, going back to the pretrial hearings. I try to have a question about the trial when I call "Talkback". My Dad helped me create some giant greeting cards for most of the major holidays and delivered them personally to the studio.

In conversation with my father several months ago, co-anchor Bill Sharpe spoke very highly of my persistence in calling them, my enthusiasm and appreciation of their efforts, my questions (which he regarded as informative and intelligent) and said that "they" meaning the key anchors had decided to "Adopt" me because as Bill Sharpe put it, "Nicky has insinuated himself into our lives here at Channel 5".

It has been and is a good experience for me. I have some help at certain times, but the major portion of my relationship with the folks at TV-5, I have done myself. I look forward to my call-ins on "Talkback" and more visits to the studio. It is a world I'd love to be a part of—and insofar as I'm able—I feel I am a part of it!

By: Nicky Weeber

Thoughts And Feelings I Shared With Bobby

To begin with many of you will notice that this isn't professional typing nor is it the greatest in the world. However, I knew Bobby better than anyone and therefore I have a few things to say about him.

To start with he loved and adored all of our family and our family pets. There were many of them—Muncho (a tiger striped cat), plus Sparky (a Labrador retriever), Sean (an English Springer spaniel), Myron and Felicia (both buff-colored cats) and adorable, and yes of course, Max (a black and white cat) with a personality all his own! Max was loved by our family and friends and was a companion to both of us up until his passing on 4/3/93. (The same day that Bobby died!)

Bobby absolutely enjoyed typing on the typewriter and sending letters to many of the daytime stars, plus watching the daytime soaps on our 19" color TV and watching movies and Star Trek episodes on the VCR. He was very interested in the soaps and that includes prime time dramas like Dallas, the Cosbys, Dynasty, Knots Landing & Falcon Crest, plus many other classic dramas and comedies.

Like myself, he grew tired of many shows, but stuck with the ones of greater quality such as Quantum Leap, L.A. Law, Murphy Brown, Murder She Wrote, Matlock and many others. He enjoyed our correspondence with many of our friends from TV and also thought the world of such people as Bill Kirk, Mary Lehman, Steve Beach, Jim Stine, Hal and Ruth Wertz from York, PA, Kathryn Beck from Elizabethtown, PA, Andy Myers and parents from York, PA, Grace Jefferson from San Diego, CA, Ike and Janie Vail from Harleyville, SC, our older sister

Wanda, Warren and Katie from Jacksonville, FL and our uncle Armin from Jacksonville, FL, and our younger sister Mary and husband John, with our new nephew (whom Bobby never saw), Joshua.

Here in Summerville we both enjoyed being visited by Dr. Bob Tapp, Dr. Buddy Craig, Dr. Ed Moore and Dr. Chip Summers—four gracious and caring gentlemen. Also, our barber, Jay Williams, came and cut our hair every month or so and we enjoyed chatting and joking with him.

When we were physically able years ago, we enjoyed shopping and going to the movies. What happened to Bobby, when he became paralyzed seems unfair and the pain he suffered was unbearable as anyone can imagine. He knew of my pain and I knew of his.

I must say that Bobby had a lot of great stories to tell and jokes. He started a story for Dr. Summers which I will soon finish.

Bobby also though highly of many nurses' aides which we had—Clara and Gloria and our newest one, Tammy. He also had high regard for the nurse, Pat, who came to see him regularly. Bobby became very fond of a special aide in a local nursing home named Alonzo who now lives in New York State. All of the people mentioned in some way or other contributed to making Bobby's life a little better. Bobby and I both found that many of the stars we wrote have a sincere love and compassion for those of us who are physically handicapped and in pain. Some of these are Bryan Buffington and Gregory Burke (2 boys we love very much and appreciate their friendship). Also, Doug Davidson, Laura Lee Bell, Kate Linder, Don Diamond and Melody Thomas-Scott from The Young and The Restless, and Matthew Ashford of Days of Our Lives. Bobby thought a lot of all of his sister Mary's girlfriends—Vicki, Lynn, Sally, Paula, Jane and Amy. He loved Mary's dog, Chianti and her cat, Verdi.

The world, as I see it, will never be the same without Bobby and Max. I know he would love my new cat, Marlena. She is very affectionate and sleeps with me at night.

Bobby often agreed with me that a lot on TV wasn't necessary and displayed a negative image for young people and we both felt that our choice of shows proved we knew more about quality TV than a lot of people gave us credit for.

He was a brave boy and a fighter, but he still was only human and deserved a better life than the one he got.

THE END!

Nicholas (Nicky) Weeber

April 29, 1993

SERVICE OF DEDICATION

In memory of
Robert V. "Bobby" Weeber
February 18, 1994

"Then God said, 'Let the earth put forth vegetation; plants yielding seed, and fruit trees of every kind on earth that bear fruit with the seed in it.' And it was so. The earth brought forth vegetation; plants yielding seed of every kind, and trees of every kind bearing fruit with the seed in it. And God saw that it was good." (Genesis 1:11, 12)

We gather here this morning to dedicate this tree to the glory of God and in loving memory of Bobby Weeber, our son, our brother, our friend. We plant this tree as a symbol of life and vitality in thanksgiving for the life and vitality of Bobby. May the rains fall gently on it, and the breezes caress it, and the sun make it grow.

Let us pray. Gracious God, who has given us this day and this tree, we present ourselves to you asking that we be allowed to worship you. Let us give thanks to you for Bobby and for his life, for the warmth and wit and laughter that were his, for the courage and patience and love that he demonstrated. We offer to you, O God, our loneliness and our tears as sacrifice for the life that is now completed. Let us give thanks to you, O God, that you have provided the resurrection of Jesus Christ for Bobby and for us. We rejoice that he lives fully in your presence, free from pain and disability, awaiting the day when we shall be reunited with him.

Now bless us on our way. Be present with us day by day as we live the life you have given us. Protect us from despair and bitterness. Open us to faith, and patience, and hope. Continue to bless Bob, and Jane, and Nicky as only you can. Accept us and our worship by the righteousness that is Jesus Christ. AMEN.

Benediction: May the love of God the Father, and the presence of God the Son, and the peace of God the Holy Spirit be with us today and forever more.

Note: The above "Service of Dedication" was delivered to commemorate the planting of a Savannah Holly tree on the grounds of Summerville Presbyterian Church in Summerville, South Carolina. The service was delivered by Dr. William F. ("Chip") Summers, Jr., former minister of Summerville Presbyterian Church.

About the Author

Robert V. Weeber has been involved in writing and publishing since 1948. He was Editor/Publisher of The Florida Funeral Director. He has also worked for newspapers as Advertising Representative and in printing sales that required copy-writing skills. He currently resides in the Summerville Presberian Home, recovering from a heart attack, suffered in the Fall of 2001.

0-595-21698-6